369 0246517

D1628610

Public Mental Health

Global Perspectives

MONKLANDS HOSPITAL
LIBRARY
MONKSCOURT AVENUE
HAIRMYRES HOSPITAL ML60JS
EAST KILBRIDE

Public Mental Health

Global Perspectives

Edited by Lee Knifton
and Neil Quinn

Open University Press

BARCODE NO: 3690246517
CLASS NO: WA 100 KNI
PRICE: 21.99
DATE: 16/7/13

Open University Press
McGraw-Hill Education
McGraw-Hill House
Shoppenhangers Road
Maidenhead
Berkshire
England
SL6 2QL

email: enquiries@openup.co.uk
world wide web: www.openup.co.uk

and Two Penn Plaza, New York, NY 10121-2289, USA

First published 2013

Copyright © Lee Knifton and Neil Quinn, 2013

All rights reserved. Except for the quotation of short passages for the purpose of
criticism and review, no part of this publication may be reproduced, stored in a
retrieval system, or transmitted, in any form or by any means, electronic,
mechanical, photocopying, recording or otherwise, without the prior written
permission of the publisher or a licence from the Copyright Licensing Agency
Limited. Details of such licences (for reprographic reproduction) may be obtained
from the Copyright Licensing Agency Ltd of Saffron House, 6–10 Kirby Street,
London EC1N 8TS.

A catalogue record of this book is available from the British Library

ISBN-13: 978-0-33-524489-8 (pb)
ISBN-10: 0-33-524489-0 (pb)
eISBN: 978-0-33-524490-4

Library of Congress Cataloging-in-Publication Data
CIP data applied for

Typesetting and e-book compilations by
RefineCatch Limited, Bungay, Suffolk
Printed and bound by CPI Group (UK) Ltd, Croydon, CR0 4YY

Fictitious names of companies, products, people, characters and/or data that may
be used herein (in case studies or in examples) are not intended to represent any
real individual, company, product or event.

MONKLANDS HOSPITAL
LIBRARY
MONKSCOURT AVENUE
AIRDRIE ML60JS
01236712005

The McGraw-Hill Companies

Praise for this book

"The book provides a convincing account of the many ways in which our society could become more mentally healthy. It should be read by businessmen, teachers and politicians as much as by clinicians."

Professor Lord Layard, Emeritus Professor of Economics at the
London School of Economics, UK

"I welcome this book as an important contribution to a pressing worldwide public health issue: how can we improve the public's mental health? The book presents work from a range of well known authors and commentators in a well structured and accessible way. It underlines the importance of the need to raise awareness of mental health right across health and wider society; finds ways of getting the evidence of what works for people and communities acted upon in more places and at a greater scale; pursue more vigorously the research agenda in public health to support improved mental health and increase our efforts in workplace mental health and employment. This book will be an extremely helpful resource for a wide range of public health professionals and many others from a range of disciplines and interests. It is important reading and represents a good example of what 21st Century Public Health needs to embrace and show leadership for. It is an important and timely contribution to a national and global challenge; one that requires new thinking and new ways of acting."

Dame Professor Sally Davies, Chief Medical Officer

"Whether you are struggling with the policy or with the practical implications of the assertion 'no health without mental health' (HM Government, 2011) this book is essential reading. Promoting mental health and wellbeing, preventing mental illness, enhancing the lives of people with mental health difficulties and what works in public mental health across the lifespan, are addressed by an international multi-disciplinary group of authors in a critical and accessible manner. The result is an authoritative, comprehensive analysis of public mental health and a wealth of practical tips for mental health clinicians, like me, on how to move their practice beyond a focus on individuals with mental illness and their families."

Professor Ian Norman, Florence Nightingale School of Nursing & Midwifery,
King's College London, UK

"This book is written by renowned experts from a wide range of disciplines who carefully explore issues and tensions within the field. It will be a great resource not just for those working in public health practice but also for all those whose work has an influence on this vitally important aspect of human life."

Professor Lindsey Davies, President of the Faculty of Public Health

Contents

List of tables

List of figures

About the contributors

John Ashton, CBE, is Director of Public Health for Cumbria and Visiting Professor of Public Health Policy and Strategy. Having specialized in Psychiatry, John became a general practitioner before moving into public health in the 1970s. Believing that practitioners should have clean minds and dirty hands, his work has straddled academia and bureaucracy, from neighbourhood through to international levels, including leading a World Health Organization (WHO) Healthy Cities Project. In 2006 he returned to the front line as Director of Public Health and Medical Officer for Cumbria, where he focuses 30 years' experience into making a difference for a population of 500,000 in a mixed urban and rural environment. He now feels that his life has come full circle with the increased recognition of the importance of public mental health. Recent work with John McKnight at Evanston University, has led him to describe ABCD as the $E=(MC)^2$ of health, complementing the recognition of the importance of focusing on outcome measures, such as sense of coherence, locus of control and self-esteem, rather than traditional biological measures that overemphasize the contribution to health and wellbeing of formal healthcare systems.

Jane Barlow, DPhil, FFPH (Hon), is Professor of Public Health in the Early Years at University of Warwick Medical School, and Director of Warwick Infant and Family Wellbeing Unit (WIFWu), which undertakes research and training in innovative evidence-based methods of supporting parenting during pregnancy and the early years. Her research focuses on evaluating the effectiveness of parent support interventions during the perinatal period, and she has also undertaken extensive research on the effectiveness of interventions in the field of safeguarding and child protection – she was an author on a recent Lancet international review of 'what works', has recently co-authored a book about 'what works' in the treatment of child emotional abuse, and a monograph for Research in Practice entitled 'Safeguarding in the 21st Century: Where to now?' She is a member of the *Early Interventions* subgroup for the Munro Review (2011), and was a member of the Department for Children, Schools and Families (DCSF) Safeguarding *Messages from Research* panel (2010). She is a sub-editor for the Cochrane Developmental, Psychosocial and Learning Disorders Review Group.

Annette L Beautrais is a Senior Research Fellow in the Faculty of Medical and Health Sciences at The University of Auckland, New Zealand, and has spent almost 20 years working in suicide research in New Zealand. During this time she has also worked in the Department of Emergency Medicine at Yale University School of Medicine. Her research interests include: psychological autopsy studies of suicide and suicide attempt; restricting access to means of suicide; suicide clusters; postvention services for families bereaved by suicide; emergency-medicine-based suicide research interventions and national suicide prevention policy and strategies. Dr Beautrais has written a large number of research papers and reviews about suicide, and has won international awards for her suicide research.

Peter Byrne is a Consultant Psychiatrist at Newham University Hospital in East London. For most of his professional life, he has worked with people with psychosis, their families and health professionals to reduce the morbidity and early mortality associated with schizophrenia.

He set up and ran two early intervention psychosis teams in London and has published on evidence-based treatments of psychosis. In addition to the psychotherapeutic modalities that characterize excellent early intervention, he has 22 years' experience of patient information/education individually and in groups (some call this psychoeducation), and using similar strategies in the wider public. He was appointed Director of Public Education for the Royal College of Psychiatrists in 2007. Dr Byrne's principal research interest is the stigma of mental illness and the effects of prejudice and discrimination on people with mental health problems. He co-wrote a textbook of psychiatry with his wife Nicola, based on the principles of problem-based learning: *Clinical Cases Uncovered: Psychiatry* (Wiley-Blackwell, published in August 2008).

Sandra Carlisle's background lies in medical social anthropology and sociology applied to public health. She has been involved, over the years, in numerous health-related research and evaluation projects. She joined the public health section of Glasgow University in February 2006 to work on a six-year research project investigating the influence of 'modern culture' on mental health and wellbeing. Long-standing research interests include: sociological and anthropological approaches to understanding health and social inequalities; community development and partnership work; community participation in action research; and ethnographic and theory-focused methodologies applied to research and evaluation. Sandra Carlisle is currently a Research Fellow at the Rowett Institute for Nutrition and Health at the University of Aberdeen.

Mima Cattan was appointed Professor in Public Health (Knowledge translation) at Northumbria University in 2009, having previously been a Reader in Health Promotion (Healthy Ageing) and Co-Director of the Centre for Health Promotion Research at Leeds Metropolitan University. Professor Cattan's research interests focus on the promotion of mental health and wellbeing in older people, mental health promotion, and the development of health promotion interventions to alleviate social isolation and loneliness in later life. From 2008 she held a part-time secondment with Folkhälsan in Finland to support the development of mental health promotion research. She has acted as expert advisor on a number of European projects on mental health promotion, and is currently a member of ROAMER, a European consortium to develop a comprehensive, consensus-based roadmap for mental health research in Europe.

Elaine Church is a Consultant in Public Health currently working across NHS Cumbria, UK. Elaine trained in psychiatry before undertaking the Masters in Public Health and membership of the Faculty of Public Health. She has a special interest in public health and mental health issues and has worked previously on the development of a mental wellbeing toolkit and national suicide audit toolkit.

Cary L Cooper is Distinguished Professor of Organizational Psychology and Health at Lancaster University, UK. He is Chair of the Academy of Social Sciences (comprised of 44 learned societies in the social sciences, representing nearly 87,000 social scientists) and President of the British Association of Counselling and Psychotherapy (37,000 members). Professor Cooper was the lead scientist on the UK government's Foresight project into Mental Capital and Wellbeing, which not only influenced policy in the UK but also in other European Union (EU) countries. He is editor of the journal *Stress and Health* (Wiley-Blackwell), and is the author/editor of over 100 books and 400 scholarly articles in the field of stress and mental wellbeing. He was awarded a Commander of the British Empire by the Queen in 2001 for his contribution to occupational health.

Patrick W Corrigan is Distinguished Professor and Associate Dean for Research in the College of Psychology at the Illinois Institute of Technology. Prior to that, he was Professor of Psychiatry and Executive Director of the Center for Psychiatric Rehabilitation at the University of Chicago. He is a licensed clinical psychologist setting up and providing services for people with serious mental illnesses and their families for more than 30 years. Ten years ago, he became principal investigator of the Chicago Consortium for Stigma Research, which evolved into the National Consortium on Stigma and Empowerment (NCSE), supported by the National Institute of Mental Health (NIMH). Central to NCSE is the Center on Adherence and Self-Determination; Professor Corrigan is the principal investigator. Located at the Illinois Institute of Technology, the Center includes co-principal investigators from Yale, Pennsylvania, Temple and Rutgers. Recent studies have examined the stigma of mental illness endorsed by employers in Beijing, Chicago and Hong Kong, through to evaluating anti-stigma programmes meant to help enlisted personnel returning from Iraq and Afghanistan, and veterans, seek out services for post-traumatic stress. He is a prolific researcher having published 11 books and more than 250 papers. He is editor of the *American Journal of Psychiatric Rehabilitation*.

Phil Hanlon was educated in the West of Scotland and graduated in medicine from Glasgow University in 1978. Following a period of clinical experience in adult medicine and general practice he took up a research post with the Medical Research Council in the Gambia, West Africa. On returning to the UK he completed a period of training in public health after which he was appointed to the post of Director of Health Promotion for the Greater Glasgow Health Board. In 1994 he became a Senior Lecturer in Public Health at the University of Glasgow and was promoted to Professor in 1999. Between January 2001 and April 2003 Professor Hanlon undertook a secondment to establish the Public Health Institute of Scotland before returning to full-time academic life as Professor of Public Health at the University of Glasgow.

Eva Jané-Llopis heads Health Programmes at the World Economic Forum. She is a specialist in health promotion and mental health, with expertise in policy-making, evidence development, implementation and evaluation of public mental health, having worked over the years in leading positions with academia, government, the European Commission and the WHO. She has led large EU research projects and think tanks, is a member of several advisory boards, has been keynote speaker in major international conferences, has published extensively on mental health and wellbeing, mental disorder prevention and public health and has led the development of networks and initiatives including the World Economic Forum Workplace Wellness Alliance.

Anthony F Jorm is a Professorial Fellow at the Melbourne School of Population Health at the University of Melbourne and a National Health and Medical Research Council (NHMRC) Australia Fellow. His research focuses on public knowledge and beliefs about mental illnesses, and particularly on interventions to improve the public's helpfulness towards people developing mental illnesses. Professor Jorm is the author of over 500 publications and has been awarded a Doctor of Science for his research and elected a Fellow of the Academy of Social Sciences in Australia. He is the chair of the Research Committee of Australian Rotary Health. He is a past President of the Australasian Society for Psychiatric Research. He has been listed in ISI highlycited.com as one of the most cited researchers in psychology/psychiatry of the past 20 years.

Lee Knifton is a Senior Research Fellow in the School of Applied Social Sciences at The University of Strathclyde. He is Deputy Editor of *The Journal of Public Mental Health*, and has recently led European-wide public health studies on stigma and workplace health. He has published widely on public mental health, stigma and equalities. He combines his academic role with practice in the National Health Service and previously in a national non-governmental

xviii   Contributors

organization developing research and policy projects. He has led a series of community-based participatory research projects on mental health with marginalized communities. He founded and directs the Scottish Mental Health Arts and Film Festival, which has grown from a grassroots event in 2007 to become one of the largest international mental health campaigns – each year engaging hundreds of organizations and over 15,000 members of the public. This work has received significant media attention and has been presented at WHO and European Commission conferences and an EU/US summit on social inclusion and transformation of mental health services.

Gregory Luke Larkin is Professor in the Department of Emergency Medicine at Yale University, and The Lion Foundation Chair of Emergency Medicine, The University of Auckland, New Zealand. He is an experienced investigator in clinical emergency medicine, biostatistics, bioethics, injury control, and mental health aspects of emergency medicine including suicide, disaster medicine and psychosocial responses to trauma, intimate partner violence and stress. He has advanced training in engineering, public health, biostatistics, research design, and has published on the psycho-epidemiology of emergency department visits for mental health problems in general and suicide in particular. Dr Larkin is Chair of the International Association for Suicide Prevention's (IASP) Task Force on Emergency Medicine and Suicide. He is a current recipient of the American Foundation for Suicide Prevention's (AFSP) Distinguished Investigator Award.

Crick Lund is an Associate Professor and Director of the Alan J Flisher Centre for Public Mental Health, Department of Psychiatry and Mental Health, University of Cape Town. He is currently Chief Executive Officer of the PRogramme for Improving Mental health carE (PRIME), a Department for International Development (DFID) funded research consortium focusing on the integration of mental health into primary healthcare in low-resource settings in Ethiopia, India, Nepal, South Africa and Uganda. He trained as a clinical psychologist at the University of Cape Town and was subsequently involved in developing norms for mental health services for the national Department of Health. He has also worked for the WHO, on the development of the WHO Mental Health Policy and Service Guidance Package, and as a consultant in Lesotho, Namibia, Indonesia, South Africa and Zimbabwe on mental health policy and planning. His research interests lie in mental health policy, service planning and the relationship between poverty and mental health in low- and middle-income countries.

Jane Mathieson studied medicine in France and qualified as a specialist in endocrinology and reproductive health in 1990. During her training, she became increasingly aware of the impact on health of social, economic and political factors, and left France to work internationally for Medecins du Monde and Oxfam, managing humanitarian relief and development programmes in Southern and Central Africa. From 2000, she has worked in Cumbria, currently as consultant in public health working with the mental health commissioning team. Her ongoing interests are public mental health and suicide prevention, health inequalities, the broad determinants of health and global health issues.

Margaret Maxwell is Professor of Mental Health and Deputy Director of the Scottish Government Chief Scientist Office funded Nursing, Midwifery and Allied Health Professions Research Unit (NMAHP RU) at the University of Stirling. Within the NMAHPRU she is the programme lead for quality and delivery of care research and Head of the Scottish Primary Care Mental Health Research and Development Programme. Within the wider School of Nursing, Midwifery and Health at the University of Stirling, she chairs the mental health, wellbeing and learning disabilities research group. She has been involved in health services research for over

25 years, focusing primarily on quality and delivery of primary care services and the management of common mental health problems, including the promotion of self-care and social interventions as management strategies.

Maura A Mulloy is currently living in Ethiopia, and is writing a book on resilience-building in schools. She received her PhD in educational psychology from the Catholic University of America in 2008, and then completed a two-year post-doctoral fellowship with the University of Maryland's Center for School Mental Health – where she divided her time between conducting research and providing mental health counselling for students in a Baltimore City elementary-middle public school. Her research interests include school-based resilience processes, the social and emotional foundations of academic success, positive psychology and strengths-based education, and mindfulness-based cognitive therapy. She is a member of the American Educational Research Association and the American Psychological Association, and earned a dissertation research award from the American Psychological Association's Educational Psychology division in 2007 for her dissertation entitled: *Still I Rise: How an Urban Public Charter High School Fosters Students' Resilient Development in Academic, Social, and Emotional Dimensions.*

Michael Nash is Lecturer in Psychiatric Nursing at Trinity College, Dublin. He is interested in professional education relating to physical health issues in mental health service users. His research and academic work covers areas such as physical care training needs analysis, mental health nurses diabetes care skills, propositional knowledge of physical health, physical adverse drug reactions and management of obesity and weight gain. He has written a book on physical health and wellbeing for mental health professionals. His current research is exploring service users' experiences of diabetes and their views of diabetes education and training for mental health nurses. Other academic and research interests include clinical risk assessment and risk management and investigating civic participation and social inclusion of mental health service users through voting.

Mary O'Hagan was a key initiator of the mental health service user movement in New Zealand in the late 1980s, and was the first chairperson of the World Network of Users and Survivors of Psychiatry between 1991 and 1995. She has been an advisor to the United Nations and the World Health Organization. Mary was a full-time Mental Health Commissioner in New Zealand between 2000 and 2007 where she had responsibility for the Commission's recovery and anti-discrimination work. Mary is now an international consultant in mental health and developer of PeerZone – recovery based workshops led by and for peers. She has written and spoken extensively on user and survivor perspectives in many countries, and has been an international leader in the development of the recovery approach.

Inge Petersen is Professor in the School of Psychology at the University of KwaZulu-Natal. She received her PhD in the field of community mental health from the University of Cape Town. Her research foci include mental health promotion and risk reduction in youth as well the development of models of community mental healthcare for scaling up mental health services in low- to middle-income countries. She is first editor and co-author of the book *Promoting Mental Health in Scarce-Resource Contexts*: *Emerging Evidence and Practice.*

Kate E Pickett is a Professor of Epidemiology at the University of York. She studied physical anthropology at Cambridge, nutritional sciences at Cornell and epidemiology at Berkeley before spending four years as an Assistant Professor at the University of Chicago. She co-authored *The Spirit Level*, with Richard Wilkinson and together they have formed the Equality Trust, which seeks to explain the benefits of a more equal society and campaigns for greater income equality.

Neil Quinn is a Senior Lecturer in the School of Applied Social Sciences at the University of Strathclyde. He has 20 years' experience in social work, community development and public health and leads a major health equity programme in one of Europe's areas of highest deprivation. His areas of expertise lie in the area of mental health, human rights and migration and he has published widely on culture and health, health inequalities, community development and participatory research with groups and communities. He leads on a number of important national and international programmes and chairs a range of groups including the Faculty of Public Health Mental Health Committee and the national Sanctuary programme working with asylum seekers and refugees. He has recently completed an EU-wide study and toolkit on depression stigma and he is co-authoring *The Implementation and Monitoring Handbook* for the *United Nations (UN) Guidelines for the Alternative Care of Children*.

Nicola J Reavley is a Research Fellow at the Melbourne School of Population Health at the University of Melbourne. She is a Chief Investigator on the MindWise project, which aims to evaluate the effects of a multifaceted mental health literacy intervention in further education students. She has experience in conducting community mental health surveys and is the Principal Investigator on two projects that aim to assess expert consensus on the appropriate strategies to include in policy and practice guidelines, one for tertiary education institutions to support students with mental illness and the other for organizations supporting employees returning to work after an episode of anxiety or depression.

Nicolas Rüsch works as a Consultant Psychiatrist and Clinical Researcher at the Department of Social and General Psychiatry, Psychiatric University Hospital Zürich, Switzerland. He trained in general adult psychiatry and neurology at the University of Freiburg, Germany and in Rome. He spent two years of research on mental illness stigma with Pat Corrigan at Chicago, focusing on how people with mental illness perceive and react to discrimination, including implicit processes, in-group perception and the impact that stigma has on service use.

Jude Stansfield is a public health specialist based in the North West of England and specializing in mental health and wellbeing. She has over 18 years' experience working locally, regionally and nationally to progress effective public mental health policy and practice. She is currently working for the Cheshire and Merseyside Public Health Network and NHS Cumbria and has undertaken work for several national organizations including the Local Government Group, the New Economics Foundation and the Department of Health.

Sarah Stewart-Brown is Professor of Public Health at Warwick Medical School, University of Warwick. She joined the University in 2003 from the University of Oxford where she had been directing the Health Services Research Unit. Her research interests focus on two areas of public health practice: public mental health and child public health. Her publications relating to parenting have played a key role in the development of parenting support policy in the UK. She continues to investigate the impact of parenting on public health particularly mental health and research interventions to support parenting. Her most recent contributions lie in the development and validation of measures of mental wellbeing for public health use. Prior to starting her academic career Professor Stewart-Brown worked in the UK NHS both in paediatrics and in public health so she brings a wealth of practical experience as well as experience in research and teaching. She has published extensively including a book on *Child Public Health* (Oxford University Press 2010). She holds a Doctor of Philosophy Degree from Bristol University and is a fellow of the UK Faculty of Public Health, the Royal College of Physicians of London and the Royal College of Paediatrics and Child Health.

Mark D Weist received a PhD in Clinical Psychology from Virginia Tech in 1991 and is currently a Professor in the Department of Psychology at the University of South Carolina. He was on the faculty of the University of Maryland School of Medicine (UMSM) for 19 years where he helped to found and direct the Center for School Mental Health (http://csmh. umaryland.edu), one of two national centres providing leadership to the advancement of school mental health policies and programmes in the USA. He has led a number of federally funded research grants, and has advised federal and national research and policy oriented committees. He helped to found the International Alliance for Child and Adolescent Mental Health and Schools (INTERCAMHS). Professor Weist has edited four books, with two in progress and has published and presented widely in the school mental health field and in the areas of trauma, violence and youth, evidence-based practice and cognitive-behavioural therapy. With colleagues from the Clifford Beers Foundation and the UMSM, he has started the new journal – *Advances in School Mental Health Promotion* (see www.schoolmentalhealth.co.uk).

Richard G Wilkinson has played a formative role in international research and his work has been published in ten languages. He studied economic history at the London School of Economics before training in epidemiology and is Professor Emeritus at the University of Nottingham Medical School and Honorary Professor at University College London. He is best known for his book with Kate Pickett, *The Spirit Level*, and together they have formed the Equality Trust (www.equalitytrust.org.uk).

Acknowledgements

We would like to thank the authors for their valuable contributions. In addition we would also take the opportunity to thank Peter Byrne, an encouraging and insightful collaborator, Andrew Kendrick for his support, and David Donald whose knowledge and advice have influenced us over many years.

We would like to thank The Royal College of Psychiatrists for permission to use the article: Kate E. Pickett and Richard G. Wilkinson (2010) Inequality: an underacknowledged source of mental illness and distress. *The British Journal of Psychiatry*, 197: 426-428. © The Royal College of Psychiatrists.

Introduction

Lee Knifton and Neil Quinn

Improving the public's mental health and wellbeing is one of the most important, contentious and exciting issues in contemporary public health. Important because international evidence increasingly demonstrates that mental health and illness has a significant impact upon population morbidity, mortality and health disparities. Contentious because concepts of mental health and illness, and agreeing what counts as evidence, are all highly political and contested. But ultimately exciting because improving public mental health and wellbeing, and reducing disparities, stimulates and necessitates new ways of thinking about public health priorities and approaches. It creates dialogue and debate across traditional boundaries and sectors and encourages interdisciplinary partnerships and communities of practice. Exciting also because despite these challenges there is an emerging consensus on public mental health priorities and an increasing evidence base about what works.

Current interest in public mental health has been driven by a number of interconnected social and public policy trends. International policy towards community-based care has ensured that mental illness has received increasing public and professional attention, and that associated issues such as stigma, discrimination and human rights became public health concerns. The increasing interest in preventing mental illness has been driven by wider socioeconomic concerns such as the costs of healthcare to the economy. Equally, although positive mental health and wellbeing have always been core concerns of philosophers and social scientists, debate on public mental health has been energized within the public health community as economic growth and prosperity has failed to deliver improved mental health or reduce overall health disparities.

Having worked as public mental health practitioners and academics for many years, we have been excited to see how this topic has been transformed from a neglected issue to a policy priority at local, national and international levels. In Scotland, for example, we have a long-term national programme for mental health and wellbeing that has adopted a public health approach entitled 'Towards a Mentally Flourishing Scotland'. This programme spans mental health and illness, drawing together a wide range of disciplines and partners, and aims to reach into and inform wider public policy and welfare provision beyond health. This trend is mirrored internationally. Thus, whereas even a decade ago the core readership of this book might have been limited to students, academics and practitioners in disciplines such as public health, health promotion, medicine and nursing, the upsurge in interest makes it just as relevant to policy-makers, social scientists, psychologists, allied health professionals and social workers.

To do justice to the scope and complexity of public mental health we have drawn upon a range of perspectives. We have brought together the collective knowledge and expertise of leading international academics and practitioners from a wide range of disciplinary backgrounds related to public health and mental health. Each chapter focuses upon a significant contemporary issue and provides an authoritative overview of that area – an expert in that area outlines the key issues and provides evidence-based direction for further research, programmes and policy. Our chapters address questions at the heart of public mental health, for example how do we prevent suicide, reduce stigma and discrimination, measure positive mental health or decide what interventions to implement in schools or workplaces? At the end, we have encouraged authors to be provocative and to share their opinions and positions on ideas and approaches that are often contested, such as the balance between social determinants and individual agency. In addition at the end of chapters you will find useful resources, tips and tools that you can use to inform and enhance research and practice in real-life situations.

To ensure the usefulness of this book, the structure and content was developed in consultation with policy makers and practitioners. This was important because the public's mental health and wellbeing can be conceptualized and addressed in a wide variety of ways. The approach we have adopted is to divide the book into four parts. In the first three parts we examine, sequentially, the promotion of positive mental health and wellbeing, the prevention of mental health problems and then approaches to enhancing the lives of people with mental health problems. This structure not only provides a useful frame of reference for understanding the major demarcations in public mental health, it is also in line with the frameworks used by many national and international programmes. This is followed by a fourth part that adopts a life-course approach and provides strong evidence about what works in bringing these public mental health approaches together in the major areas of childhood and parenting, schools and adolescence, adult working lives and later life.

We begin with 'promoting positive mental health and wellbeing', an area that pushes the traditional boundaries of public health. In Chapter 1, Phil Hanlon and Sandra Carlisle call for a new public health approach. They challenge the notion that economic growth in itself is sufficient to maximize overall population wellbeing or to reduce disparities. Drawing upon historical and interdisciplinary ideas they highlight the interconnectedness of local and global efforts. In Chapter 2, Jane Mathieson and colleagues develop the idea that 'community' is central to enhancing the mental health and wellbeing of individuals, families and groups. Against a backdrop of increased social isolation and reduced community cohesion in more affluent nations (Putnam 2000) and increased economic disparities within and between countries, they focus upon the importance of socioeconomic regeneration and community development approaches. Inge Petersen and Crick Lund then provide a very comprehensive overview of evidence-based approaches to promoting mental health and wellbeing in resource-scarce countries. Drawing upon their experience they highlight both the similarities and differences as compared with higher-income countries. They discuss the importance of addressing basic needs and what we can learn from public health work with other health conditions. Despite the challenges of combating poverty and meeting basic needs they stress that there is no health without mental health, even, or especially, when resources are very limited. They also highlight that there are lessons to be learned across countries. Finally Sarah Stewart-Brown provides a valuable examination of the ways in which we can measure positive mental health and wellbeing, which is vital if we are to understand and progress our collective knowledge of what works. Acknowledging different philosophical and political positions, and drawing upon evidence from across disciplines, she rebalances the debate by stressing the importance of agency, and not just structure, in how we consider, respond to, and measure positive mental health.

The second part of the book tackles the challenge of preventing mental health problems. Prevention is driven by the public health burden associated mental health problems (World Health Organization (WHO) 2008) and also the major economic costs of healthcare treatment and loss of productivity (Dewe and Kompier 2008). Our opening two chapters highlight two approaches to prevention that draw upon different public health traditions. In Chapter 5, Kate Pickett and Richard Wilkinson argue that relative-income inequality is the main predictor of mental health and associated problems. It provides a compelling argument that for meaningful prevention of mental health problems we need to concurrently address social conditions and structures. The public health challenge is to work to develop policies and programmes that reduce this disparity, or which prevent the widening of the gap. In Chapter 6, Nicola Reavley and Anthony Jorm instead focus upon a public education approach to prevention. They examine the evidence that increasing overall individual and community knowledge (or 'literacy') about mental health problems can reduce prejudice and increase aspects such as help-seeking and community support. Mental health literacy forms a central part of many national public mental health programmes and the authors highlight useful resources and implications for practice. In Chapters 7 and 8 Annette Beautrais and Gregory Luke Larkin focus upon suicide prevention and Margaret Maxwell focuses upon preventing depression. Depression and suicide are two of the most significant public health problems that we face. Data from WHO predictions on the global burden of illness have placed depression as the second leading cause of disability worldwide (Murray and Lopez 1997). Each year an estimated one million people worldwide die by suicide, the leading cause of violent deaths, and in some countries the third leading cause of death among 15- to 44-year-olds (WHO 2012). This makes a focus on prevention imperative and each chapter provides an impressive and comprehensive overview of the extent of the nature and the extent of the problem as well as evidence-based interventions in an international context. But what is equally important is that they highlight the sociocultural contexts of mental health and illness, the deficiencies in existing approaches and potential new directions.

The third part of the book focuses upon enhancing the quality of life, and the wellbeing, of people who live with a diagnosed mental health problem. We focus upon recovery, stigma and discrimination, early intervention and physical health. The health and equality of people with mental health problems are not just the concerns of mental health practitioners and service user/consumer organizations but of the wider public health community. The numbers of people with mental health problems, and the impact upon people's lives of a diagnosis, makes this a public health, and an equalities, priority. Our opening chapters on recovery and stigma are written by internationally leading authors, and can be considered in the context of wider civil rights struggles. They are about social justice in public health. In Chapter 9, Mary O'Hagan draws upon her personal and professional experience and provides a compelling case for a reorientation of services and communities towards a recovery ethos and approach. She introduces an historical perspective, challenges illness constructs and highlights power differentials. She then provides a framework and resources for both practitioners, policy makers and commissioners to help make this happen. Importantly, these ideas inform and have been informed by approaches to promoting wellbeing for the whole population. We then focus upon how we can tackle stigma and discrimination in Chapter 10. Whereas many national public health programmes have tried to tackle stigma and discrimination through social marketing and public education approaches, Nicolas Rüsch and Patrick Corrigan argue for a more evidence-based, sophisticated approach. In particular, they stress the central role of positive contact. Then, drawing upon their internationally renowned work, they outline promising practice and case studies. Peter Byrne, in Chapter 11 then provides a strong rationale for the development of services that intervene early with people who are at risk of developing psychosis. He argues that we must offer flexible approaches to engage and support young people at risk. In addition to providing evidence for the need and effectiveness of this model, he draws upon his experience to provide guidance on how to implement an early intervention service in practice. Finally, in Chapter 12, Michael Nash outlines the poor physical health outcomes of many people with long-term mental health problems. He addresses the underlying causes of this, including institutional stigma, and suggests how we can reduce this health inequality.

In our final part we bring together the ideas that have been developed throughout the preceding three parts on promotion, prevention and quality of life. Leading authors highlight how to 'bring it all together' through a life-course approach. In doing so we recognize that very often the actions that promote positive mental health, prevent mental health problems or promote quality of life can be interlinked. Our four chapters focus less upon developing specific projects but instead on harnessing community and non-mental health organizations to achieve maximum improvement in public mental health. In Chapter 13, Jane Barlow demonstrates why early years are a critical point influencing future mental health and provides clear guidance on how parenting interventions can work. In Chapter 14 Maura Mulloy and Mark Weist then provide an evidence-based framework that can be used to promote, prevent and support the mental health and wellbeing of young people, in partnership with school staff, as part of a whole school model. This is especially important given that many mental health issues arise in childhood and adolescence and that school settings enable population-scale interventions. In Chapter 15, Eva Jané-Llopis and Cary Cooper build the case for prioritizing workplaces. Work is generally beneficial to mental health at a population level and for most people with enduring mental illnesses, provided it is fair and well supported. It is also the main mechanism by which income is (re)distributed in societies. They make both a business and a public health case for prioritizing workplaces, especially in the current economic climate. Aptly, our final chapter is about later life. Mima Cattan highlights the extensive and often neglected problems of poor mental health in later life including social connectedness, physical and mental health and poverty in later life.

As you progress through the chapters you will see a great deal of consensus, and optimism, among the authors. However, a number of interesting tensions and debates are also apparent that we explore in the final chapter (Chapter 17). We hope that you find this book stimulating, provocative and practically useful.

Part I
Promoting positive mental health

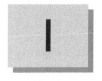

Positive mental health and wellbeing: connecting individual, social and global levels of wellbeing

Phil Hanlon and Sandra Carlisle

Introduction

The burgeoning science of positive mental health and wellbeing contains much that is of value for the public health community. Although definitions vary, positive mental health is generally seen as including emotion (affect/feeling), cognition (perception, thinking, reasoning), social functioning (relations with others and society) and coherence (sense of meaning and purpose in life). All these are important for individual wellbeing and a growing number of longitudinal studies confirm their power to predict outcomes such as longevity, physical health, quality of life, drug and alcohol use, criminal behaviour, employment, earnings and pro-social behaviour, such as volunteering (Friedli 2009). Such findings have inspired optimism about the role of positive psychological attributes in enabling people to flourish, notwithstanding adverse circumstances, and have led to a renewed interest in therapies that focus on transforming how people think, and how they think about their lives (Seligman 2002; Diener and Seligman 2002; Frederickson 2005). The new discipline of positive psychology is a clear leader in this field. Yet its focus remains strongly individualized and, from a public health perspective, in need of balancing with evidence and insights from other relevant sources (Carlisle and Hanlon 2008). This chapter therefore attempts to draw together knowledge and evidence from the many disciplines that bear on mental health and wellbeing at individual, social and even global levels. Inevitably, given the size and scale of this task, we have had to oversimplify much, and we ask our readers to view this chapter as a brief overview of some extremely complex territory.

The first section of the chapter explores the relationship between positive mental health and wellbeing, constructs that have been shown by research to be closely related but not entirely interchangeable. The following sections provide a brief synthesis of some key strands of theory and evidence about what influences individual wellbeing, much of which derives from the discipline of psychology and its modern variant, positive psychology (Seligman 2002).

Limitations of the latter are briefly highlighted. Later sections draw on more critical knowledge from other behavioural and social sciences, which needs to be taken into account in understanding the evolutionary, social, economic and cultural context that shapes and influences mental health and wellbeing (Carlisle and Hanlon 2007). Economics, for example, has an extensive history of research interest in wellbeing and recent thinking from this discipline challenges long-held assumptions in Western society about what creates wellbeing. Sociologists have observed that the increasing individualism and materialism, associated with the modern economy and its consumer culture, undermines wellbeing at individual and social levels. Expanding the analytical lens still further, emerging environmental changes now call into question the sustainability of our current way of life, while widening inequalities across the world threaten human health and wellbeing at the global scale. The broad perspective taken in this chapter leads to a perhaps unexpected conclusion: what makes for good mental health and real wellbeing is, ultimately, as much a matter of social justice as one of individual psychology. The chapter ends with a few examples of practical action to promote wellbeing, together with some suggestions as to how such activities might be evaluated, followed by a number of key reflection points and questions for the reader.

The relationship between positive mental health and wellbeing

According to research by Keyes (2002), the absence of mental illness does not necessarily imply the presence of high levels of positive mental health. Conversely, he has found that people with mental health problems may also experience positive mental health. Within the discipline of psychology, positive mental health is more usually recognized as a combination of subjective wellbeing (or positive feelings) and good (positive) psychological functioning (Huppert 2005). This understanding integrates two distinct philosophical approaches to the definition of wellbeing, both of which can be traced back to the philosophers of Ancient Greece (Ryan and Deci 2001). The hedonic perspective on wellbeing emphasizes feelings of pleasure or happiness, whereas the eudaimonic perspective emphasizes engagement, fulfilment and meaning or purpose – conceived in ancient philosophy as the good or virtuous life. In contemporary research, these two perspectives are often termed subjective wellbeing and psychological wellbeing.

However, researchers in the field have observed that positive feelings by themselves are not sufficient for good mental health as these may be transitory, achieved in unsustainable ways (through alcohol or drugs, for example) and do not necessarily lead to personal fulfilment. Moreover, there will be occasions in most human lives where the experience of negative feelings is normal and part of good mental health, such as grief for the death of a loved person (Williams 2000). On the other hand, positive mental health and wellbeing cannot be achieved solely by realizing one's potential or living a life of virtue, because contentment and joy are also a vital part of the good life, the life worth living (Csikszentmihalyi 2004). On this basis, subjective wellbeing (or happiness) should not be dismissed as a trivial or frivolous issue. The science of positive mental health and wellbeing therefore often combines a focus on satisfaction with life, overall happiness and good psychological functioning. For people to be able to experience the condition of 'flourishing', they need to feel satisfied with their lives, that they are developing personally and that they function positively in regard to their society. Research suggests that the experience of life satisfaction is strongly related to good mental health and inversely related to depression – all of which is relevant to the public health community, given the global increase in mental health problems such as depression and anxiety (WHO 2001a). Equally relevant, research also suggests that a sense of ongoing personal development relates well to overall health, longevity, resilience and the ability to cope with adverse circumstances and thrive in life (Singer and Ryff 2001).

Nevertheless, for the public health community, the individualized focus of much psychological research on mental health and wellbeing may reduce its significance. Huppert (2005), however, has argued for an epidemiological perspective that recognizes how broader risk factors at play in society influence our mental health and wellbeing. She draws on the work of Geoffrey Rose (1992) to suggest that the most effective way of reducing the prevalence of mental ill health is to shift the mean of the population in a beneficial direction, towards greater mental health and wellbeing, by reducing the risk factors. A small shift in the prevalence of mental distress across the normal distribution would result in a large shift in the tail of the distribution. In other words, more people would flourish – or at least enjoy moderate mental health – and fewer would languish, or experience mental disorder and distress. Yet the question of 'risk' and 'protective' factors for wellbeing is extremely complex, as we need to think about these at both individual and social levels. This issue weaves its way through the remaining sections of this chapter.

Is a 'positive psychology' sufficient for mental health and wellbeing?

An extensive body of research now suggests that psychological assets confer resilience and protection at both an individual and an ecological level (Bartley 2006). Optimism, self-esteem, self-efficacy and interest in others are characteristics of resilient adults, neighbourhoods and communities, where norms of trust, tolerance, support, participation and reciprocity may provide some protection from the effects of deprivation (Friedli 2009). However, a number of critics have also pointed out that a focus on positive thinking and feelings may lead to a disembodied psychology, which separates people's thoughts and feelings from their social structure and cultural context (Friedli 2009). A key therapeutic intervention then becomes to change the way people think, rather than to tackle the key catalysts for psychological problems such as money worries, poor housing, degraded urban environments, lack of opportunity, violence and crime. A corrective to the 'change the way we think' position is to understand that our values and the ways in which resources are distributed in society (e.g. by economic and fiscal policy) are key domains that influence and are influenced by how people think, feel and relate.

A growing body of international data shows strong contextual effects for material factors. For example, people at the same level of income will have lower mortality if they experience more, rather than less, equal states (Wilkinson and Pickett 2010). One explanation for this (and for the strong social gradient in health) is that relative deprivation is a catalyst for a range of negative cognitive and emotional responses to inequity. These are both conscious and unconscious reactions, influencing health through physiological reactions, through the impact of low status on identity and social relationships (Bourdieu 1984), as well as through a range of damaging behaviours that are a direct or indirect response to the social injuries associated with inequalities (Rogers and Pilgrim 2003). In this analysis, levels of inequality have a strong impact on how people feel, and those feelings are powerful but persistently underestimated indicators for good or poor mental health. This suggests that our individual and collective mental health and wellbeing may actually depend on reducing the gap between rich and poor, rather than on promoting individual-level interventions such as cognitive behavioural therapy (CBT).

What influences wellbeing?

A number of influences on wellbeing have been suggested by psychological research. Some, for example, have suggested that we all have a genetic predisposition to a certain level of happiness (Lykken 1999), sometimes referred to as a 'set point'. It is also the case that certain personality traits such as optimism and extraversion tend to be associated with greater wellbeing. Another key influence on wellbeing is life circumstances: income, material possessions, marital status, neighbourhood and so on. For some psychologists, however, our circumstances are believed to count for less than heredity, as research has demonstrated that humans are extremely adaptable to circumstances, whether positive or negative (Brickman et al. 1978; Kahneman 1999). This suggests that, although people in our society tend to spend much of their time on seeking to improve their life circumstances, such efforts may be wasted, if improving their sense of well-being is the ultimate goal (Nesse 2005). Yet another key influence on wellbeing is provided by our 'intentional activities' – pursuits we actively engage in (such as socializing, exercising, working towards life goals and so on) and cognitive activities (such as appreciating life). Because such activities are varied and impermanent we do not adapt to them, which prompts researchers to suggest that this may be the area where improvements in wellbeing can be most easily achieved.

Other factors that impact on wellbeing should also be mentioned, albeit briefly. For example, unemployment has been found to be a major source of unhappiness, but good quality work is an important source of wellbeing. Physical health also matters strongly for individual well-being, although people's objective health status appears less relevant than how they perceive their condition. The discipline of positive psychology has also provided evidence of what works in promoting mental health and wellbeing (Lyubomirsky 2010), such as learning to dispute overly negative interpretations of our selves or our life situation, being grateful for what goes well in life, appreciating those important to us, and practising altruistic behaviour and kindness towards others. Developing appropriate coping strategies for adverse circumstances has also been found effective in protecting mental health and wellbeing (Lyubomirsky 2011).

Turning now to the discipline of economics, basic thinking here has long assumed that people are 'rational actors' who promote their own wellbeing (or 'utility') by exercising free choice in life, which in turn is facilitated by income. However, researchers in this discipline have found that increases in income and economic growth contribute little to average levels of wellbeing across society, *once basic needs are met* (Easterlin 1974; Lane 2000). Research conducted over many decades shows that those of us who live in affluent countries seem not to feel any better about our lives, despite rising living standards and incomes (Lane 2000; Schwartz 2004; Layard 2005). Yet economics has also persistently found richer people in such countries to be happier than their less-well-off peers. How are such apparently paradoxical findings to be reconciled? What really seems to matter for wellbeing is the increase in social status that a larger income brings, not the money itself (because we readily adapt to this). Thinking from evolutionary psychology echoes this point, in that human males are believed to be 'hard-wired' to seek social status, as this improves their chances of finding a mate and reproducing (Nesse 2005). We are thus burdened with a positional psychology that derives from our evolutionary heritage, past the point where it conferred sufficient advantage in wellbeing terms: 'stone-agers living in the fast lane', to use the oft-quoted title of a well-known paper (Eaton et al. 1999).

Much research confirms that we are all socially comparative beings: we compare ourselves with a range of people, and this affects our sense of wellbeing for good or ill – a point that illustrates the limitations of considering positive mental health and wellbeing as primarily an individual matter. Wellbeing is ineluctably a product of the interplay between individual, community and social influences and factors (Haworth and Hart 2007). Overwhelmingly, the largest message of the whole body of wellbeing research is that we should pay far more attention to fostering good relationships with others, and less to increasing our standard of living (Marks and Shah 2005). Pleasurable feelings and experiences matter for our subjective wellbeing, certainly in the short term, but good relationships with others helps to protect and promote our mental health and wellbeing over the longer term, whether these take the form of marriage or other intimate partnership, family networks, close friendships or a supportive community and social network (Layard 2005). Yet, an emerging body of research suggests that these funda-mental elements of wellbeing are undermined by certain aspects of modern society that encourage us to stay on the hedonic treadmill, in pursuit of short-term happiness.

Wellbeing: a casualty of modern society?

Few would deny that late modern societies have benefited from economic growth, despite the existence of persistent health and social inequalities. Yet, over recent decades a number of prominent sociologists (Lasch 1979; Featherstone 1991; Beck 1992; Bauman 2001) have high-lighted the interdependence between an increasingly globalized capitalist economic system, contemporary cultural traits such as individualism, materialism and consumerism, and declining levels of individual and social wellbeing (Carlisle et al. 2009). These arguments are echoed in some public health research (such as Eckersley 2006). Contemporary consumer culture appears to corrode individual character and undermine social solidarity and resilience (Sennett 2006), while modern economic conditions dictate that people work in a far less secure atmosphere (Bauman 1998). Traditional working class culture, which helped provide a sense of solidarity in the past, has virtually disappeared whereas the 'new' middle classes appear highly individualized and increasingly isolated from any sense of community (Rutherford 2008).

It has been observed that the materialist desires of many people in contemporary culture undermine any deeper sense of purpose and meaning in life (Schwartz 2000; James 2007). Meanwhile, the search for happiness in consumer products and services props up the modern economy but produces little in the way of genuine wellbeing (Hartmut 1998). Standardized consumption patterns, promoted through advertising, become central to economic growth while consumption becomes a substitute for the genuine development of the self (Giddens 1991). People construct their social identity via their consumption choices (Ransome 2005) but this is fraught with risks around making the 'wrong' choices in life. For the poor of affluent society, faced with limited choice, life can be particularly difficult and individuals can be spurred into debt in order to avoid shame (Lury 2003). In sum, modern society is associated with the emer-gence of an individualized, materialist, consumer culture in which confidence and resilience are undermined at individual, community and social levels (Bauman 1998). Although the evidence-based strategies of positive psychology may help the individual to develop positive ways of coping (such as Frederickson 2005), they cannot address the social and political nature of the problems outlined here. The observed trend towards values and practices that erode confidence, resilience and general wellbeing at individual and social levels thus point to the importance of finding alternative ways of finding meaning and purpose in life (Hanlon and Carlisle 2009).

The bigger picture: global problems and social justice

Evidence and thinking from diverse fields is now converging in a shared concern about the long-term, global consequences of the increasingly dominant – and globalized – cultural system associated with the Western way of life. The increasing obsession, in 'modern' society, with superficialities such as wealth, fame, physical appearance and material possessions is linked not just to the decline of care and concern for others in the world but to the neglect, even potential destruction, of humankind's shared environment (Cafaro 2001). From this perspective, continued overconsumption by the few may ultimately render the physical world uninhabit-able for all. A broad conclusion, supported by steadily accumulating evidence from the environ-mental sciences (Intergovernmental Panel on Climate Change 2007), is that the dominant cultural norms and values found in many Western-type societies have resulted in a marked imbalance between a specific way of life and the planet's environmental carrying capacity (Harrison 1993).

Humanity faces looming global changes as at least a partial result of this imbalance. These include anthropogenic climate change (McMichael et al. 2006), which could lead to multiple socioeconomic impacts such as mass migration and many public health challenges. We may now have passed the peak in oil production (Hubbert 1945; Roberts 2005): the loss of this energy resource on which many depend will inevitably lead to dramatic social change on a global scale, with implications for health and wellbeing. It is therefore not surprising that psychological researchers Ryan and Deci (2001) warn that, as individuals pursue satisfying and pleasurable aims within affluent societies, they may create conditions preventing the attainment of wellbeing by others. These writers urge attention to the relationship between personal wellbeing and broader issues such as the collective wellness of humanity and the planet. In similar vein, Csikszentmihalyi (2004), one of the founders of the positive psychology movement, argues that we need a new image of what it means to be human: the efforts of those living in modern societies to create comfortable environments, in the belief that this will improve life, have undermined the essence of what makes life worth living over the long run.

Taken together, these arguments suggest that modern Western societies need to reconsider some deeply held assumptions about how we should live (Hanlon and Carlisle 2009). The idea of the good life – the life worth living – returns us to the importance of wellbeing in both its subjective and psychological forms. If it is plausible that good mental health and wellbeing enable people not just to survive difficult times, such as the current global recession, but also to thrive, then greater attention to this dimension of human life and health is both warranted and increasingly urgent. Conversely, increasing compassion for others and concerns for the environment (and the physical limits to resources) have the potential to counter trends towards materialism, individualism and consumerism, and in so doing could also contribute to our health and wellbeing, as individuals and social beings on a finite planet.

Mini toolkit

We have outlined some daunting challenges above. We end this chapter with two very different illustrations of what can be done in practical terms to improve mental health and wellbeing, at individual and wider levels. The first example below briefly describes a set of five evidence-based actions that are being used by various organizations to promote mental health and wellbeing at community level. The second example is a community-based response to the social injuries of modernity and the resulting loss of meaning and purpose in many lives: the GalGael Trust, which is a charitable organization based in the former shipbuilding area of Govan in Glasgow. The examples are followed by some suggestions as to how such initiatives can be appropriately evaluated.

Tips for effective practice

The centre for wellbeing at the New Economics Foundation (nef) was commissioned, by the UK Government's *Foresight* programme (Mental Capital and Wellbeing Project, The Government Office for Science 2008) to develop a short set of actions that individuals could use to improve their personal wellbeing (Aked et al. 2008). By drawing on an extensive evidence base of 'what works', nef concluded that five ways to wellbeing could be recommended for individual use.

- We should all try to connect with those around us – family, friends, neighbours, work colleagues as these connections provide the cornerstone of wellbeing in our lives.
- We should try to be physically active – much evidence shows how important this is for wellbeing, within the limits of our own fitness and mobility.
- We should take notice of and appreciate the things around us, savour the moment and reflect on our experiences and feelings.
- We should keep learning throughout life – new skills, hobbies and so on.
- We should give to others and practise kindness, understanding that our own wellbeing is connected to those around us.

More information and the full report are available at: www.neweconomics.org/projects/five-ways-well-being.

Various examples of the ways in which these actions have been given practical form at community level can be found in the case studies published on the Local Government Development and Improvement website: www.idea.gov.uk.

Case study: The GalGael Trust – navigating life

The relentless decline of the ship-building industry in Govan, on Scotland's Clydeside, left many in that community bereft of work and purpose in life. Like many other post-industrial areas left behind by the fast-flowing current of modernity, mental health problems and various kinds of addiction emerged. The founders of the GalGael Trust understood that such problems are related to the loss of identity and the sense of meaninglessness that creates vulnerability to the worst excesses of modern life, all of which are worsened by the consistent undermining of the bonds of community. The GalGael Trust provides a cultural anchor point around which both a sense of purpose in life and a shared sense of kinship and community are re-kindled, while the slide towards a dependency culture is resisted.

The Trust is trying to change the perceived drudgery of modern work by renewing its roots in the heart of the community. The method used, at its workshop in Fairley Street, Govan, is deceptively simple: provide people with a place to work, some basic respect, and with tools both practical and attitudinal. A practical part of GalGael's success is that participants are taught artisan skills using natural materials like wood, wool and stone. At a deeper level, participants themselves told us that, in working on reclaiming and transforming wood, they were simultaneously working on reclaiming and transforming their own lives. The results are patterns of learning and productivity that are capable of reshaping shattered identities and filling empty lives with creativity, purpose and worth. For more information, see the Trust's website at: www.galgael.org.

Undertaking research and evaluation

There is great pressure on many practitioners to evaluate the effectiveness of their interventions. One problem here is that there is a gap between the contemporary rhetoric of evidence-based policy and practice, and what happens on the ground, which is known to be far more complicated (Coote et al. 2004). For example, community-based wellbeing programmes are rarely designed to deliver a single intervention with one specific goal: they can be made up of a wide range of activities and projects, and draw on different fields and knowledge bases. In this context, evaluation is widely recognized as challenging (Raphael 2000).

Participation, the use of multiple methods, the goal of local capacity building and appropriateness of method have all been suggested as key principles that should underpin the evaluation of any community-based initiative, in order to accommodate their complex nature and potential longer-term impact. In particular, the turn to participatory forms of research reflects a growing interest in the recapture of forms of knowledge that have been excluded from many conventional forms of enquiry.

One approach to evaluating community-based wellbeing initiatives is participatory action research (Carlisle et al. 2007). Participatory action research attempts to counter the powerful currency of academic research by valuing the contribution that local people can make to the shared development of knowledge, and also develops that knowledge to inform action and construct evidence. This approach to evaluation thus rejects the traditional research view of non-academic participants as repositories from which data can be extracted, and the evidence generated is firmly grounded in local research and practice.

Another approach is that provided by theory-based approaches to evaluation (Weiss 1995; Pawson and Tilley 1997). These take for granted that all health and/or social programmes are based on explicit or implicit 'theories' about what is believed will work in producing hoped-for outcomes. Theories used in this sense are not remote abstractions but common-sense, practical ideas and beliefs. Theory-based evaluation stresses that theories underpinning any initiative should be spelt out at an early stage in the wellbeing intervention, so participants understand their overall goals and can specify how to achieve these. Project theories then become the 'test' by which projects can be evaluated.

Neither of these approaches is without its own difficulties. There is also the point that those on the receiving end of the evidence derived from such initiatives cannot be viewed as empty vessels waiting to be filled with information before taking policy and/or practice decisions. The usefulness of evidence generated through the various forms of knowledge produced through the approaches suggested above still remains contingent on key public sector agencies' and policy makers' capacity and willingness to learn from – and be convinced by – the product. On the other hand, although it can be difficult to specify cause-and-effect relationships within a community-based initiative seeking to promote wellbeing, an emphasis on process and on community members and participants' perceptions and interpretations, makes their detection more likely.

Reflection points and questions

- The question of 'risk factors' for mental health and wellbeing is extremely complex. The discipline of positive psychology has focused on developed therapies that focus on transforming how individuals think and feel about their lives. Such findings need to be balanced with research and thinking that helps us understand how other influences (evolutionary, social, economic, political and cultural) also have a role in shaping individual and social health and wellbeing.
- The 'modern' trend towards values and practices that erode confidence, resilience and general wellbeing at individual and social levels points to the importance of finding alternative ways of finding meaning and purpose in life. A key message from wellbeing research is that we need to foster good relationships with others, rather than increase our standard of living, as the search for happiness in consumer products and services props up the modern economy but produces little in the way of genuine wellbeing.
- Inequality threatens wellbeing at many levels. Levels of social inequality impact strongly on how individual people feel about their lives and those feelings are powerful indicators for good or poor mental health and wellbeing. Global inequalities threaten not just the sustainability of the 'modern' way of life but the health and wellbeing of all humankind.

- These points prompt a number of questions. If a focus on individual psychology and social/global justice are important in creating good mental health and real wellbeing, how may we as individuals seek fulfilment, joy, engagement and purpose in life? In the context of an unequal (and possibly unsustainable) society, how can we best promote these things for, and with, others? And how should we judge the effectiveness of our actions? We do not have the answers: these questions are for all of us to consider.

Further reading and resources

The arguments we have outlined over the course of this chapter are explored in greater detail in a new website (www.afternow.co.uk). We have developed this as a learning resource for the broad public health community and others interested in wellbeing. In a series of videos, audio files and downloadable papers we describe the challenges we all face in creating and promoting health and wellbeing in modern society. The site has seven major sections:

- a 'change of age';
- the 'dis-eases' of modernity;
- the threat of collapse;
- new ways of thinking, being and doing;
- navigating the journey to a sustainable future;
- in search of transformational change.

Other useful sources and resources include:

- Huppert, F., Bayliss, N. and Keverne, B. (eds) (2005) *The Science of Wellbeing*. Oxford: Oxford University Press. This is a multidisciplinary text that documents key findings and insights into the determinants of good mental health and wellbeing and how these may be promoted.
- Haworth, J. and Hart, G. (2007) *Wellbeing: Individual, Community and Social Perspectives*. Basingstoke: Palgrave MacMillan. This book usefully emphasizes the interplay between social, community and individual wellbeing and the importance of a global perspective on this issue.
- Friedli, L. (2009) *Mental Health, Resilience and Inequalities*. Copenhagen: World Health Organization Europe. This report makes important connections between mental health and inequalities. Like Haworth and Hart, Friedli focuses on promoting resilient individuals, communities and environments.
- Last but certainly not least, numerous research-based and policy-relevant reports on wellbeing and how it may be promoted at individual, social and global levels are available from the website of the new economics foundation (www.nef.org.uk).

2 | Community development, regeneration and mental health

Jane Mathieson, John Ashton, Elaine Church, Jude Stansfield and Neil Quinn

Introduction

In this chapter we consider the extent to which community development and regeneration policies, programmes and initiatives have the potential to have a positive impact on mental health and wellbeing. In so doing, we explore some of the challenges in evaluating this impact, in particular the diverse understandings of, and theoretical approaches to, community development and regeneration, and the limited availability of high-quality evidence. Notwithstanding these limitations, and given the compelling evidence of an association between social and material living conditions and population mental health, we go on to examine which approaches to community development and regeneration may have the greatest potential to improve mental health and wellbeing outcomes. We focus particularly on approaches that empower, contribute to individuals' and communities' 'sense of coherence', and recognize their inherent capabilities and assets.

We locate this discussion within the turbulent context of contemporary Britain. We explore some of the characteristics of public policy drivers influencing the community development agenda, in particular, disinvestment in the public sector and policies promoting localism under the banner of the 'Big Society'. Within these constraints, we explore the recent emergence of assets-based approaches. We also suggest that community development should embrace its radical origins and empower citizens to critique policies and interventions that may have a negative impact on mental health and wellbeing.

We conclude with a section of 'top tips' from our own practice, suggesting how to embed asset-based community development approaches as an integral part of the policy and practice framework to improve mental health and wellbeing and reduce inequalities in mental health.

Definitions and key concepts

Mental health and wellbeing are subjective experiential processes intrinsic to each of us as individuals, they are located within a web of interactions and relationships with others. This conceptualisation is consistent with current debates about the fitness for purpose of the WHO's definition of health as complete wellbeing. Huber and colleagues (2011) have proposed a change of emphasis towards the ability to adapt and self-manage in the face of social, physical and emotional challenges. These definitions are also consistent with Antonovsky's Salutogenesis model (Antonovsky 1979; Lindstrom and Eriksson 2005). Elaborated in the 1970s, this model has re-emerged in current debates about what supports health and wellbeing, rather than what can precipitate disease.

The term 'community' is an evolving concept and definitions of community are elusive, imprecise, contradictory and controversial (Popple 1995). While acknowledging this, 'community development' has been defined as 'the process of assisting people to improve their own communities by undertaking autonomous collective action' (Twelvetrees 2008: 1). Within community development, there is an explicit concern to make the existing system work better for those who are marginalized from society (Alinsky 1972).

The term 'regeneration' is used to refer to a wide spectrum of physical, economic and/or social policies and interventions, from improvements to the housing stock and transport infrastructure, to opportunities for training and employment and improved delivery of health and social services. Some form of community development is often, but not systematically, a feature of regeneration initiatives.

Theoretical frameworks underpinning community development and their relationship to health outcomes

Theory has played an important part in shaping trends in community development practice. Arnstein's (1969) ladder of participation describes eight levels of citizen participation from tokenism to control, underpinned by the aspiration towards a redistribution of power across society. Paolo Freire's *Pedagogy of the Oppressed* (1972) was highly influential in the domains of community development and community health as well as in education. Linking the identification of issues to positive action for change and development, Freire set the framework for a radical approach to collective mobilization. Similarly, Robert Chambers' experience of community development in developing countries led him to conclude that successful and sustainable outcomes can only be achieved when experts and professionals give up power and control over project outcomes to the people directly affected by them (Chambers 1997).

Within the USA 'community organizing' is also seen as a process by which people are brought together to act in common self-interest, helping people recognize that they face shared injustice and can work together to overcome this (Rubin and Rubin 2008). Community organizing for health is underpinned in the following concepts (adapted from Minkler and Wallerstein 2005).

- Empowerment: promoting a social action process whereby individuals, groups and communities gain mastery over their lives in the context of changing social, economic and political circumstances.

- Critical consciousness: undertaking a social analysis of living conditions and people's role in changing these conditions.
- Community capacity: building the ability of communities to identify, mobilize and address public health problems.
- Social capital: developing the structures and relationships that facilitate coordination and cooperation for mutual benefit.
- Issue selection: identifying winnable and specific targets of change that unify and build community strength.
- Participation and relevance: ensuring that community organizing starts where people are and engages community members as equals.

Community organizers enable social movements by building a base of concerned people and mobilizing people to act. Building community is seen as a means to increase social justice, individual wellbeing and reduce the negative impacts of otherwise disconnected individuals.

Asset-based community development is an approach that, like the salutogenesis model, focuses on individuals' and communities' resources and capabilities rather than deficits or needs, and aims to empower communities to take control of these assets. This approach, developed extensively by John McKnight in the USA, identifies and builds upon the assets of local citizens and communities (Kretzman and McKnight 1993). This ethos has a long tradition within mental health through the strengths-based perspective, which focuses on the resilience and strengths of communities and their hopes for the future (Saleeby 2006). Although the assets-based approach is critiqued for its tendency to minimize the role of the welfare state in delivering health and other outcomes, and to emphasize self-help, it has resonance in contemporary Western societies in the context of contracting health and social care budgets.

The theoretical framework outlined in Figure 2.1 usefully summarizes these considerations (Popay 2010). It hypothesizes that different levels of community engagement could directly and indirectly affect health in both the intermediate and longer term. Approaches that relocate more power and control to communities may lead to more positive health outcomes and may also improve other aspects of people's lives, for example, by improving their sense of belonging to a community, empowering them, encouraging health-enhancing attitudes and behaviour or otherwise improving their sense of wellbeing.

Thus, empowerment is both a desirable outcome in itself, and also potentially an intermediate step towards improved health status and greater equity in outcomes (see also Wallerstein 2006).

The evidence base linking community development and regeneration approaches to improved mental health, wellbeing and resilience

There is compelling epidemiological evidence of the links between social and material living conditions, mental health and mental illness (Rogers and Pilgrim 2003). As highlighted in the recent Marmot Review (Marmot 2010), and *No Health without Mental Health* (Department of Health 2011a), social and economic inequalities are damaging to mental health and wellbeing; and mental illness is often associated with stigma and multiple disadvantage. Conversely, resilient communities have lower levels of crime and violence and higher levels of pro-social behaviour and social integration/relationships. Resilient individuals have more fulfilling relationships, lower prevalence of physical as well as mental illness, and higher educational achievement, employability, productivity and earnings (Friedli 2009).

This evidence base supports the intuitive assumption that interventions that have the potential to alleviate socioeconomic deprivation and increase community and individual

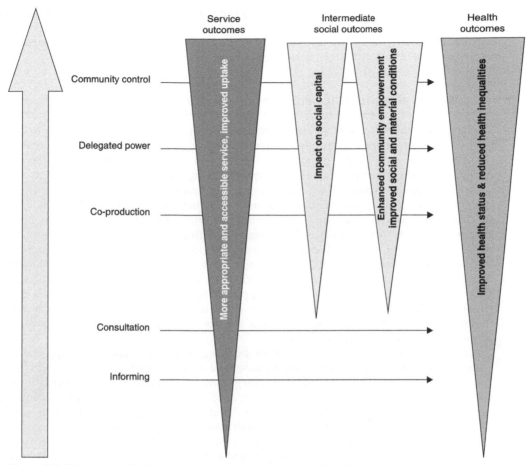

Figure 2.1 The relationship between community engagement and health outcomes.

resilience – including community development and regeneration initiatives – could lead to improved health. A range of social and economic, as well as health, benefits could potentially accrue to communities as a whole and to individuals involved as recipients or providers of such initiatives. The beneficiaries of such interventions could include: communities and groups with distinct health needs; communities that experience difficulties accessing health services or have health problems caused by their social circumstances; and people living in disadvantaged areas (National Institute for Health and Clinical Excellence (NICE) 2008a).

However, there is relatively little high-quality impact data to confirm this assumption. Multiple activities are often combined in community development and regeneration initiatives and research studies and evaluations are rarely explicit about the approach used. Few studies evaluate the direct impact of particular community engagement and/or regeneration approaches on health outcomes. Improving mental health and wellbeing is even more rarely articulated as a specific outcome. Similarly, cost-effectiveness studies of community development and regeneration initiatives are hampered by the long duration of such initiatives, the difficulties in attributing outcomes to the particular approach used and difficulties in predicting what might have happened if the intervention had not taken place (Wallerstein 2006; NICE 2008a; Knapp et al. 2010).

Notwithstanding these limitations, some of the key findings reported in evidence reviews of community development, regeneration and health are outlined below.

Community development approaches and mental health

Wallerstein's international review of the evidence on effectiveness of empowerment to improve health (2006) suggested that empowering initiatives can lead to improved health outcomes and that empowerment is a viable public health strategy. In particular, coalitions and interorganizational partnerships that promote empowerment through enhanced participation and environmental and policy changes have led to a range of health outcomes including psychological empowerment. This review further suggests that empowerment is a complex strategy whose success may depend as much on the agency and leadership of the people involved, as the overall context in which they take place. For example, youth empowerment interventions can have positive health outcomes including strengthened self- and collective-efficacy, stronger group bonding, formation of sustainable youth groups, increased participation in structured activities including youth social action, and policy changes, leading to improved mental health and school performance. Engagement of young people in structured organized activities that link them to each other and to institutions can enhance their self-awareness and social achievement, improve mental health and academic performance and reduce rates of dropping out of school, delinquency and substance abuse.

A recent review of the economic case for building community capacity (Knapp et al. 2010) adds a further perspective to the evidence base. The authors' original intention was to examine the economic case for broad-based community development programmes. However, in view of the paucity of evidence of effectiveness, they focused instead on components of community development initiatives for which they considered there was sufficient evidence on which to estimate the economic benefits, namely timebanks, befriending, and community 'navigators' who provide debt and benefits advice. Based on the (albeit limited) evidence of positive impacts of these three types of interventions on physical and mental health, as well as improved social, welfare and employment outcomes, the authors concluded that they generate net economic benefits over a relatively short time period.

Within the UK the review by NICE (2008a) of community engagement approaches to health improvement found some evidence that they can have physical and mental health benefits. However, it also concluded that when done badly, community engagement can have negative health impacts. The review's recommendations emphasize certain prerequisites for effective community engagement, in particular a long-term policy commitment to invest in engagement, to build trust and respect between partners and to share power; and development of an infrastructure for, and approaches to support, engagement (NICE 2008a).

Regeneration and mental health

Thomson et al.'s (2006) review of urban regeneration programmes in the UK concluded that although health and mortality impacts were assessed, conflicting data made it impossible to draw conclusions. More recently an evaluation of the National Strategy for Neighbourhood Renewal in the UK (Department for Communities and Local Government 2010) makes little reference to health outcomes, beyond singling out worklessness interventions as having made a contribution to improved mental health.

Other work has looked more specifically at the links between housing improvement, as part of regeneration initiatives, and health outcomes. Thomson and Petticrew (2005) found robust evidence that housing improvements can have a positive impact, particularly on mental health, although regeneration has the potential to increase exclusion and divisions within an area and for those living on the margins of a regenerated area, feelings of exclusion can exacerbate levels of stress and depression. Gibson et al.'s (2011) synthesis of systematic reviews of interventions aimed at different pathways linking housing and health found that, of the seven studies that assessed mental health impacts of housing conditions, all but one reported positive effects. Further evidence of the psychosocial impacts of housing interventions has been provided by the Scottish Health, Housing and Regeneration Project (SHARP) (Kearns et al. 2008).

Another review examining the relationships between neighbourhood accessibility, social networks and mental wellbeing concluded that increased participation in formal groups and associations does not necessarily equate to increased social capital or improved wellbeing, but opportunities for informal networking in the public realm are important to people (Parry-Jones 2006).

Notwithstanding conceptual difficulties and the limitations of the evidence base, this overview suggests that community development and regeneration initiatives can impact positively on mental health, particularly through improvements in people's living and working conditions, their social interactions, and processes of empowerment. We will now go on to examine how these findings can be operationalized within policy and practice with particular reference to the context of the current UK coalition government's reform agenda.

Optimizing mental health through community development and regeneration in contemporary Britain

There is a long history of linking regeneration and community development to improve health in the UK, going back to the Pioneer Health Centre in Peckham in the 1930s (Pearse and Williamson 1938/1982). However, this focus shifted and community development has more recently gravitated from its strong early links to health, education and social work, towards economic development and regeneration. For instance, from 1997 the UK's New Labour government invested heavily in area-based initiatives such as Neighbourhood Renewal, Single Regeneration Budget and its New Deal for Communities. Housing has been a major focus of this regeneration work and the mental health impact of such programmes can be illustrated by SHARP (Box 2.1).

Box 2.1 The Scottish Health, Housing and Regeneration Project (SHARP)

This is a longitudinal study of the health and social effects on tenants of moving into new-build socially rented housing. The primary aim was to investigate the health and wellbeing impacts of being rehoused in new-build socially rented housing, with a particular focus of the study looking at mental health impacts. The study found those people rehoused experienced substantial improvements in some aspects of their mental health and wellbeing, such as status, identity and sense of progress. Before rehousing, mental health and wellbeing was worse among people living in regeneration areas than in other areas. Over time, and after rehousing, mental health and wellbeing improved more for people living in regeneration areas than in other areas, although the differences were not statistically significant. The results suggest that area regeneration can support mental health and wellbeing gains from rehousing, although the provision of houses with gardens serves to maximize the mental health and wellbeing gains from rehousing. On the other hand, the prevalence of loneliness was higher and worsened among residents in regeneration areas, indicating that area-wide disruption may affect people's sense of social integration, at least during the course of regeneration. However, loneliness was lower among people who moved into houses rather than flats, and improved more among people who reported gains in the safety, security and accessibility of their homes (Kearns et al. 2008).

Although there has been a major focus by community development on regeneration, since the advent of community care there has again been an increasing recognition that community development can have a role in promoting health, including improving mental health and wellbeing and addressing mental health inequalities in partnership with regeneration bodies. One case study that illustrates this well is the Positive Mental Attitudes (PMA) programme in Glasgow (Box 2.2).

Box 2.2 Positive Mental Attitudes: a community and regeneration programme in an area of high deprivation

Positive Mental Attitudes is a mental health inequalities initiative that has operated for ten years in East Glasgow, the UK's highest concentrated area of socioeconomic deprivation, which has developed a broad coalition of community support with mainstream funding and over 50 partners from a range of sectors including housing, education, regeneration, arts and culture, and planning agencies. The programme has built capacity within local community groups and agencies to deliver a wide range of community development initiatives ranging from school lessons and arts events to peer-led community conversation workshops. Initiatives have worked face-to-face with tens of thousands of people, and have informed national strategies and international programmes. Further information can be found at: www.positivementalattitudes. org.uk.

We are now entering a new chapter in the relationship between community development, regeneration and mental health and wellbeing. Since 2010, the UK coalition government's reform programme has been dominated by large reductions in public spending, policy changes and new ways of working within the public and third sectors, and a shift towards localism and the 'Big Society' agenda. This has led to a disinvestment in regeneration (Department of Communities and Local Government 2010). At the same time there is a strong focus in policy discourse on the concept of wellbeing. The rhetoric of the 'Big Society' draws on assets-focused approaches, interwoven with discourses of localism and wellbeing (Local Government Improvement and Development 2010). Notwithstanding these policy challenges and the widespread reservations about the Big Society, it remains the main current policy vehicle for community development. One of the drives behind the Big Society is to support local groups to provide self-help and there are a number of initiatives that focus on mental health and wellbeing. A good example of this can be found in Cumbria within the north-west of England in the development of a community support group for people bereaved by suicide (Box 2.3).

Box 2.3 A community support group for people bereaved through suicide

One of the first tasks of the Cumbria multiagency suicide prevention group, formed in 2009, was to meet members of the local mental health service user and carer association, Cumbria Mental Health Group (CMHG). Family members were able to explain how their experience of bereavement was like no other. One person's remark summed it up: 'I wish we could talk about it more'. When, later, members of CMHG were asked, through a public consultation exercise, to suggest ideas for the introduction of asset-based approaches into the county, reactions were mixed. Although mutually supportive, members did not want to find themselves signed up to 'self-help' in disguise. However, CMHG did agree to take a lead in organizing a support group for people bereaved through suicide. With the help of the national charity, Survivors of Bereavement through Suicide (SOBS), the Cumbria group has now been running for over a year. As well as meeting regularly, some members have become active advocates for suicide prevention, appearing regularly in the local media and calling on health and social care services to address the inadequacies in current statutory bereavement support provision. Also, SOBS Cumbria has received small amounts of funding from the local health authority to cover meeting and training expenses, as well as transfers of knowledge and services in kind.

Despite these opportunities within this new policy environment for community development, concomitant policies that envisage large-scale reductions in public services and welfare have led to critiques of the Big Society in terms of wider concerns about the potential impact on population mental health and wellbeing of the government's policies. Moreover many have voiced concerns that the Big Society – wrapped up in notions of assets-based community development, volunteering and social enterprise – is a pretext for shifting responsibility for local public services to local communities, with little accompanying resource and a cut in the existing infrastructure supporting community development. As such, the deployment of assets-based community development approaches may be a thinly veiled way to transfer responsibility for the delivery of certain services deemed 'non-essential' from the public to the community realm in a constrained policy environment.

However, the distinctive emphasis in all three case studies is, on the one hand, a recognition of lay people's knowledge, capabilities and assets, and ways in which these can be mobilized to enhance individual and collective wellbeing; and on the other, empowerment – a concern to equip people with the knowledge, skills and confidence in their own abilities to influence the decisions that affect their lives. When aligned to the values of radical community development, it can be a transformational tool, empowering communities to have greater control over their destinies.

Conclusions

In this chapter we have illustrated the potential for improving mental health through community development and regeneration interventions. We have suggested that asset-based approaches with a strong empowerment focus offer the most promising practice internationally. These interventions must acknowledge and build on people's inherent capabilities, assets and resources. They should increase people's awareness of what constitutes wellbeing, remove barriers to participation and equip people with the additional skills and support they need.

However, there are obvious limits to what community development and regeneration programmes can achieve in terms of mental health improvement. These interventions have limited population coverage, targeting specific communities and/or areas, and, more important, limited influence on the wider structural factors in society that contribute to social and health inequalities, as outlined in recent international and UK-based reports focusing on the social determinants of health (Commission on Social Determinants of Health 2008; Marmot 2010). The current global turbulence calls for a return to the radical roots of community development, a fertile ground where we are empowered as citizens to question and critique policy, call for equity and social justice, and act for change beyond the boundaries of our communities.

Mini toolkit

Top tips for effective practice

Assets-based community development approaches offer a very useful model to maximize the impact of community development and regeneration interventions on mental health and wellbeing. They support the deployment of available individual, community and public resources in ways that optimize mental health and other outcomes. Some of the actions underpinning this implementation of this approach are as follows.

- Promoting wellbeing as a unifying concept behind which local authorities and communities can align their efforts, ensuring that local policies, programmes and interventions support wellbeing.
- Developing empowerment strategies so that communities not only take control of local assets but also have the knowledge, skills and influence to challenge policy makers.
- Investing in resilience – especially of children and young people, through universal prevention services and targeted early intervention approaches.
- Securing sign up from local organizations to tackle the social determinants of poor population mental health, such as poverty, social injustice and discrimination.

Case studies

Examples include the following.

- The Lambeth Mental Well-Being programme, an initiative shaped by local people to make their community and neighbourhood a better place to live (www.lambethfirst.org.uk/ mentalwellbeing/).
- Integrating and embedding mental wellbeing in Greenwich, a community development initiative to improve mental wellbeing through addressing environmental factors, which has led to low-cost improvements to buildings and homes (www.nhsconfed.org/Networks/ PrimaryCareTrust/case-studies).
- The Spice Timebank (www.justaddspice.org), which enables people in an area to exchange skills and assets and has led to increased self-esteem and confidence. The Blaengarw Time Credit project in Wales has revitalized the community with over 700 people now giving their time through time banking and 34 new local groups have now been developed.

Undertaking research and evaluation

- Process is central to community development and should be evaluated alongside impact.
- When assessing impact, adopt appropriate measures that relate to the core purposes of the project – for example are you aiming to improve social conditions, social capital or the wellbeing of certain community citizens?
- Community-based participatory research has become a powerful research approach in public health by focusing upon action and equity, maximizing participation, building capacity and validating the lived experiences of marginalized communities.

Reflection points and questions

- What are the limitations and weaknesses of community development as an approach to reducing mental health inequalities?
- How do you acknowledge and minimize power imbalances when using community development approaches in public health?
- How can we build meaningful and sustainable capacity for community leadership on health issues?

Further reading and resources

- The Asset-Based Community Development Institute (ABCD): http://www.abcdinstitute. org/about/founders/.
- Foot, J. and Hopkins, T.A. (2010) *A Glass Half Full: How an Asset Approach can Improve Community Health And Wellbeing*. London: IdeA. Available at www.idea.gov.uk/idk/ aio/18410498 (accessed 21 August 2012).
- Local Government Improvement and Development (LGID) (2010) *The Role of Local Government in Promoting Wellbeing*. London: LGID. Available at www.idea.gov.uk/idk/ aio/23693073 (accessed 21 August 2012).
- North West Public Health (2010) *Living Well across Local Communities. Manchester: North West Public Health*. Available at http://www.nwph.net/hawa/details.aspx?pid=103& type=rep&id=2227 (accessed 21 August 2012).
- Foresight Mental Capital and Wellbeing Project (2008) *Final Project report – Executive summary*. London: Government Office for Science. Available at http://www.bis.gov.uk/ assets/biscore/corporate/migratedD/ec_group/116-08-FO_b (accessed 4 October 2012)
- Community development with minority communities for mental health: www.mosaics-ofmeaning.info.

3

Mental health promotion in developing contexts

Inge Petersen and Crick Lund

Introduction

Neuropsychiatric disorders account for 13 per cent of the global burden of disease and contribute 8.8 per cent and 16.6 per cent of the total disease burden in low- and middle-income countries (LMICs) respectively (WHO 2008). In the face of a treatment gap exceeding 75 per cent (Saxena et al. 2007; Kessler and Ustun 2008), there have been a number of recent initiatives targeting the scaling up of mental health services in LMICs that advocate, *inter alia*, for a task-shifting approach to address this gap (Chisholm et al. 2007; Patel and Prince 2010; WHO 2010a). Task shifting refers to the delegation of tasks where appropriate, to less specialized health workers in the provision of healthcare services under the supervision of scarce specialist health personnel.

While these scaling up efforts are important to alleviate suffering, they are unlikely to reduce the prevalence of mental disorders as new cases arise. To address this problem, mental health promotion and mental illness prevention interventions are important to reduce the incidence of new cases. Although fairly well established in high-income countries (HICs), mental health promotion and mental disorder prevention has received little attention in LMICs where the emphasis has been on the scaling up of treatment services.

Definition of mental health promotion

Mental health promotion is concerned with promoting optimal psychophysiological development and mental health in people. Mental health is defined by the WHO as: 'a state of well-being in which the individual realises his or her own abilities, can cope with the normal stresses of life, can work productively and fruitfully, and is able to make a contribution to his or her community' (WHO 2001b: 1).

The goal of mental health promotion is to achieve this state of wellbeing in all individuals. It employs various public health strategies to reduce exposure to modifiable risk factors for mental ill health as well as strengthen protective factors to promote resilience in the face of risk. In so doing, mental health promotion interventions may help to prevent, ameliorate or reduce disabilities associated with mental disorders. Although mental health promotion may overlap with the prevention of mental disorders, mental health is not just the absence of a mental disorder (WHO 2004a). Mental health promotion strives to promote effective functioning of people so as to strengthen the human capital of societies. Preventing the onset of mental disorders is the goal of primary prevention, which specifically aims to reduce the incidence of mental disorders. Early detection and treatment so as to reduce the severity of a mental disorder are the aims of secondary prevention. Rehabilitation to prevent relapse in people with mental disorders is the purview of tertiary prevention. Although mental health promotion overlaps with prevention and treatment and may use similar strategies, the outcomes are different and complementary (WHO 2004a). The focus of this chapter is on mental health promotion.

Importance of mental health promotion in LMICs

Mental health promotion is particularly important in LMICs because of the many modifiable risk factors that exist in these countries, particularly those associated with poverty. Mental illness and poverty interact in a vicious cycle that is evident across the lifespan. Poor nutrition and ill health during prenatal development and infancy can result in micronutrient deficiencies that can impair normal brain development (Walker et al. 2007b). Exposure to toxins, disease, birth trauma, poor maternal responsiveness and lack of psychosocial stimulation during infancy can result in cognitive and socioemotional deficits (Richter et al. 2010). In the absence of opportunities later in life to compensate for these early deficits, the developing person is vulnerable to being trapped in a negative cycle of poverty and mental ill health. Grantham-McGregor et al. (2007) estimate that over two-hundred million children in LMICs have impaired cognitive abilities as a result of poverty-associated malnutrition and inadequate care.

In adults, studies indicate that certain dimensions of poverty, in particular lower levels of income, education, worse housing, increased food insecurity, unemployment and financial stress are associated with common mental disorders, such as depression, anxiety and somatoform disorders (Lund et al. 2010; Patel et al. 2010). Although the causal pathways in LMICs are not well established, data from HICs suggest that the stressors of living in poverty, and associated risks such as social marginalization, exposure to violence and food insecurity may trigger the onset of common mental disorders. In turn common mental disorders result in increased health expenditure, increased cost to households as a result of caregiver time and opportunity costs, reduced productivity and ability to work, stigma, reduced access to health-care and substance abuse (Patel et al. 2010), perpetuating the cycle of poverty and mental ill health (see Figure 3.1). People with severe mental illness, who may not initially live in conditions of poverty, may also be at risk of drifting into poverty as a result of increased health expenditure, reduced productivity, job loss, stigma and increased caregiver time and related household level opportunity costs (Saraceno et al. 2005).

Physical ill health also impacts negatively on a person's mental health and vice versa (Prince et al. 2007b). This is of particular concern in LMICs given the greater burden of communicable diseases (WHO 2004b), especially HIV/AIDS which has a high comorbidity with mental disorders as a result of the psychological burden of the disease or direct effects on the central nervous system, such as HIV-related dementia (Prince et al. 2007b; Brandt 2009). In addition to depleting a person's immune system, these mental disorders can interfere with treatment adherence as well as increase risk behaviours, escalating transmission rates of HIV and other communicable diseases (Prince et al. 2007b).

Mental health promotion interventions hold potential for breaking this cycle of mental ill health and poverty, enabling more positive social and economic outcomes for the beneficiaries/recipients and thereby promoting broader socioeconomic development through

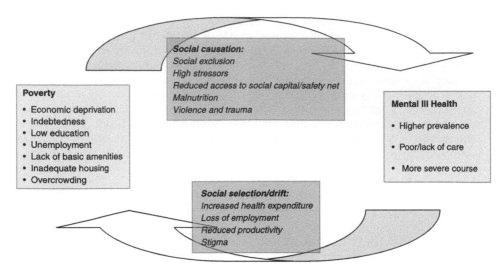

Figure 3.1 Cycle of poverty and mental ill health.

the development of the human capital asset base in LMICs. This is most clearly illustrated by mental health promotion interventions in early childhood. Long-term follow-up of beneficiaries of a protein nutrition intervention study (1969–1977) by the Institute of Nutrition of Central America and Panama (INCAP) in Guatemala found that women who had been exposed to a more nutritious supplement and had completed primary school had better educational achievement than those exposed to a less nutritious supplement (Walker et al. 2007a). Adult males who had been exposed to the more nutritious supplement from 0 to 2 years had an hourly wage rate 46 per cent higher than the average hourly wage rate of the sample (Hoddinott et al. 2008). These findings provide evidence from an LMIC of the long-term impact that a nutrition intervention in early childhood can have on moderating negative sociocontextual conditions to promote human capital development and enhance the potential for economic growth (Grantham-McGregor 2007).

Principles of practice

An ecological developmental framework

Mental health is influenced by the interplay of multiple risk and protective factors that range from distal upstream social determinants discussed above, through proximal environmental influences and life experiences at the interpersonal and community levels, to individual-level influences such as inherited genetic structure and physical health. In this context, mental health promotion interventions are best informed by an ecological framework, such as that depicted in Figure 3.2, that highlights the interdependence of risk influences operating on the development of mental ill health within the different social systems.

In addition, the impact of these risk influences varies depending on the developmental life phase of the person. Across the lifespan, there are sensitive periods in psychophysiological development when contextual influences and life experiences interact with genetic influences to affect specific developmental processes. The most sensitive period is during prenatal

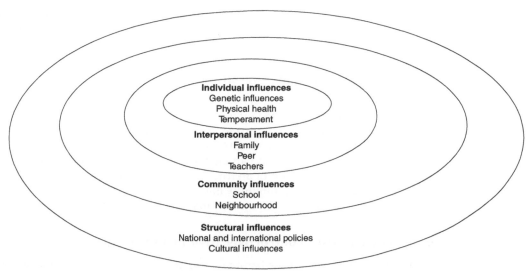

Figure 3.2 Ecological level of risk and protective influences.
Source: Petersen et al. 2010

development and infancy (1–2 years) when neural plasticity is greatest, and which gradually decreases over time. Mental ill health arises out of the interplay of multiple risk influences and a paucity of protective influences. Even though vulnerabilities in early life disproportionately affect mental health and wellbeing later in life, the trajectory towards mental ill health is not necessarily linear. Earlier vulnerabilities can sometimes be compensated for by protective factors later in life (Richter 2006; Tomlinson and Landman 2007).

As indicated in the framework, distal societal- and population-level interventions are needed to address upstream social determinants of mental disorders. This is particularly important in LMICs given that many of the risk influences for mental ill health during prenatal development and childhood, as well as in adults, are associated with conditions of poverty. These interventions are, however, not unique to mental health promotion and overlap with many public health and other initiatives aimed at combating socioeconomic inequities and promoting human and socioeconomic development.

Proximal interventions, more unique to mental health promotion, can promote positive development and mental health in the context of risk, strengthening protective factors to moderate or mediate outcomes in the context of risk. This underpins the concept of resilience, which is an important strategy for mental health promotion interventions in LMICs given greater exposure to poverty-related social determinants of mental ill health. These interventions aim to strengthen protective factors at the individual level, as well as immediate protective interpersonal and community influences.

Protective factors can be strengthened at the individual level, through altering an individual's response to a stressor, for example, by improving personal coping strategies. At an interpersonal level, strengthening protective factors, such as improving parental support, can moderate the impact of stressors on children. Parental support interacts with the stressors to moderate their impact on the child. In the absence of parental support, the impact of exposure to a traumatic event can be mediated by the introduction of a caregiver. In this case, the new caregiver plays a compensatory role, independent of the traumatic event. Strengthening social capital at a community level can also promote healthier outcomes in the face of stress. Social capital refers to the benefits accrued from belonging to social networks and includes, *inter alia*, social support and bridging social capital, which refers to access to resources (Carpiano 2006).

Ensuring cultural and social fit of programmes

Although there are many examples of effective mental health promotion interventions from HICs there is a paucity of evidence-based interventions in LMICs. Simply transporting interventions that have been found to be effective in HICs to LMICs gives no guarantee that they will be effective in these contexts (Barry 2007). Formative studies to understand the local cultural context and their needs as well as participation of community members and beneficiaries in the development or adaptation of an intervention are important to ensure ecological and cultural fit (Sperber et al. 2008). Community members themselves are best placed to provide insight and local knowledge on interventions that may mediate pathways to health.

Empowering people to have control over their mental health

Mental health promotion builds on the basic tenets of health promotion as contained in the Ottowa Charter (1986). As such, a basic principle is to promote empowerment and enhance people's control over their mental health and its determinants (Barry 2007). Empowerment occurs when people have a sense of control over their lives as well as their environment. It can be fostered through democratic participation in support groups, self-help groups and action-oriented groups where individuals may gain new skills and build social capital. This is particularly important in LMICs given the greater likelihood of exposure to poverty-related social determinants of mental ill health. Individual and collective empowerment can facilitate people taking action to address the social determinants of mental ill health – thus fostering greater individual and community control over mental health.

Theoretically driven interventions

Theories are important to inform the programme design. Mental health promotion draws on multiple theories from lifespan development theories, health promotion theories of behaviour change to theories in community and health psychology (Barry 2007). Individual- and interpersonal-level theories generally strive to strengthen protective influences to moderate or mediate the impact of risk influences, building resilience in the face of exposure to risk. With moderation, the outcome of exposure to a risk factor is moderated by protective factors that interact with a risk factor, for example, strengthening parenting skills can moderate the impact of exposure to risk influences in children. With mediation, the effects of a protective factor operate independently from a risk factor, compensating for the negative outcome of the risk factor. For example, exposing a child to a bereavement programme following the death of a parent. Theories at the community level promote empowerment of community members to take action to reduce exposure to risk influences. Theories at the societal level generally relate to policy-level changes.

Evidence-based interventions

The implementation of evidence-based programmes in LMICs is essential given limited resources that need to be used wisely and efficiently to ensure superior outcomes for beneficiaries as well as widespread reach to those in need. Evidence-based interventions are also more likely to be funded and attract resources.

Although randomized control trials (RCTs) remain the gold standard for evidence-based interventions, and should be used wherever possible, they are often difficult to implement in LMICs. This is particularly so for community-level interventions where the use of an RCT may be constrained by cost, ethical, practical and political reasons. In these instances, the effects of interventions may need to be evaluated using other designs such as quasi-experimental designs and qualitative studies (Bhana and Govender 2010).

Mental health promotion across the lifespan

Prenatal development and infancy (1–2 years)

Multiple environmental influences and experiences during the prenatal period and infancy can predispose infants to a wide variety of disorders later in life. These include *micronutrient deficiencies* especially iodine and vitamin folic acid; and *exposure to infectious diseases* that can interfere with normal neurocognitive development and cause deficits in cognition, attention and learning as well as poor socioemotional and motor functioning in children (Durkin 2002; Walker et al. 2007b; O'Connell et al. 2009). Exposure to *environmental toxins* such as lead, arsenic, pesticides, tobacco smoke and alcohol also negatively affect the developing brain, placing the developing foetus and infant at risk for cognitive deficits. *Cerebral insults* associated with birth trauma, particularly anoxia, can cause a range of mental and physical disabilities (Richter et al. 2010). *Disturbances in early infant–caregiver relationships* such as loss of primary attachment figures, caregiver depression as well as abuse and neglect can result in disturbances in social and emotional development and interpersonal attachments later in life as well as behavioural disorders, anxiety, depression and attention problems (Richter et al. 2010). *Deprivation in psychosocial stimulation during infancy* has also been found to be associated with cognitive and socioemotional impairment (Richter et al. 2010).

Many of these risk influences during prenatal development and infancy are more prevalent in LMICs, the bulk of which are modifiable. *Distal* mental health promotion interventions that are not necessarily unique to mental health promotion include public health efforts to, *inter alia*, improve the diet of pregnant and lactating mothers as well as reduce environmental toxins and improve maternal and child healthcare services to prevent obstetric complications during childbirth.

Proximal interventions unique to mental health promotion that have been shown to be effective in LMICs include selective postnatal home visitation programmes. Two examples include a programme in Jamaica that provided nutritional support and psychosocial stimulation in growth retarded or stunted infants; and a programme in South Africa that promoted maternal sensitivity and mother–infant attachment. Both interventions used trained community workers within a task-shifting approach to deliver the intervention. The Jamaican study had four groups: a control group, a stimulation only group, a nutritional supplementation only group and a combined stimulation and supplementation group. The study provides long-term comparative outcome data on cognitive and socioemotional functioning across the four groups. The nutritional supplementation was 1 kg of milk-based formula per week. The stimulation component involved community health workers improving mother–child interactions through play during weekly home visits over the two years. Over these first two years, children in receipt of both interventions showed higher levels of cognitive development than children in receipt of a single intervention. However, at 22 years, participants who received the psychosocial stimulation intervention had higher adult IQ scores, obtained higher educational attainment, displayed few depressive symptoms and reported less involvement in fights or serious violent behaviours than those individuals who did not (Walker et al. 2011).

In the South African programme, women were visited weekly, twice antenatally and then for eight weeks postnatally and then monthly for two months ending five months postnatally. The intervention aimed to sensitize mothers to their infants' needs and capacities and promote more sensitive responsive parenting through the home visitation programme. While no long-term data is available from the South African trial, the programme was able to improve maternal sensitivity in the intervention group at 12 months compared with controls and the intervention children were more securely attached than controls at 18 months (Cooper et al. 2009).

Children and adolescents

During the preschool years (3–5 years), the development of social relatedness and self-regulatory control are important developmental tasks that can be hampered by harsh and inconsistent parenting and reduced opportunities to learn pro-social skills. Failure to adequately accomplish these developmental tasks can impede children's capacity to function effectively later on within a school environment, placing such children at risk of poor school performance as well as poor peer relations, which can lower self-esteem and promote behavioural problems in school-going children. Exposure to undue stress such as child maltreatment, family conflict/violence or parental loss/separation are risk factors throughout childhood. They can result in regressive behaviours, such as bed-wetting and anxiety during the preschool years when these self-regulatory processes are still developing; as well as a range of externalizing behavioural disorders and internalizing mood and anxiety disorders in school-going children (Richter et al. 2010).

Although examples from LMICs of evidence-based mental health promotion interventions for the preschool period are sparse, early childhood programmes that combine early education with family support and parenting programmes to foster nurturing parent–child relationships have been found to have promising outcomes in HICs (Barnett 1995). Zippy's Friends provides an example of a school-based programme for the promotion of socioemotional competencies and adaptive coping skills in pre- and elementary school aged children (5–7 years) that has been successfully adapted for use in LMICs (Mishara and Ystgaard 2006).

During middle childhood (6–12 years), cognitive development continues and building self-esteem and social competence are important developmental tasks. Adolescence (10–20 years) is characterized by many developmental challenges, including puberty, the development of more abstract thought and the development of a sense of self-identity. It is noted for being a particularly vulnerable period for engaging in risk behaviour that can impact negatively on the mental health and life-course of a person (Richter 2006). Family strengthening and parenting programmes that aim to improve family relations, communication and parental monitoring have been found to promote good mental and behavioural health outcomes for children and adolescents in LMICs (Bhana 2010; Flisher and Gevers 2010). The Collaborative HIV/AIDS Adolescent Mental Health Programme South Africa (CHAMPSA) provides an example of an effective family-based intervention targeting pre-adolescents (Bell et al. 2008) that was originally developed in the USA and successfully adapted for use in South Africa using a cartoon-based narrative. The programme was delivered to multiple family groups comprising caregivers and their children over ten sessions. Given the high prevalence of HIV/AIDS in South Africa, a number of sessions were devoted to HIV knowledge and stigma and discrimination in addition to parent strengthening sessions, which included rights and responsibilities of parents and children, monitoring and control and parent–child communication. On completion of the programme, families that participated in the intervention demonstrated, *inter alia*, improved caregiver monitoring and improved caregiver–child communication compared with control families (Bell et al. 2008).

In addition to parenting programmes, school-based programmes, particularly life skills programmes have been found to be effective in both HICs and LMICs to promote socioemotional coping, particularly during adolescence when youth are particularly prone to negative peer influence. Life skills programmes in schools have been shown to be successful in improving decision-making, affect management and conflict resolution, as well as assisting to avoid peer pressure to engage in risk behaviours and connect adolescents to supportive community resources (Flisher and Gevers 2010). Whole school programmes that promote school connectedness have also been found to be promotive of mental and behavioural health, serving to buffer negative home environments, although evidence from LMICs is sparse (Bhana 2010; Flisher and Gevers 2010).

Adults and older people

Although pre-existing vulnerabilities are important risk factors for mental ill health in adults and older people, there are also a number of independent social risk factors for mental ill health that can operate independently or interact with pre-existing vulnerabilities to increase mental ill health. A number of recent reviews on the social determinants of common mood and anxiety disorders provide empirical support for certain poverty-related conditions being associated with common mental disorders in LMICs, namely, low education, food insecurity, poor housing and financial stress and low socioeconomic status relative to others (Lund et al. 2010). Exposure to stressful and traumatic events such as violence and other crimes, conflict and disasters; chronic physical ill health; and stressful working environments have also been associated with post-traumatic stress disorder (PTSD), other anxiety disorders, depression and substance abuse (Patel et al. 2010).

In addition to distal interventions to address these social determinants of mental ill health that overlap with many public health and poverty alleviation initiatives, proximal- and individual-level interventions have potential to promote mental health in LMICs. These include interventions that build social support, particularly participatory group-based interventions that combine microfinance opportunities with a critical empowerment approach. An example is the Intervention with Microfinance for AIDS and Gender Equity (IMAGE) programme in South Africa that included a microfinance intervention with a participatory learning programme that aimed to build an awareness of gendered power imbalances as well as promote confidence and communication skills. This intervention was shown to improve mental health in women, promote gender equity and reduce intimate partner and sexual violence.

The promotion of healthy lifestyles is also important during adulthood. This can assist with substance abuse problems as well as help to prevent dementia in older people. The burden of dementia is increasing in LMICs and risk influences include hypertension, type 2 diabetes, hypercholesterolaemia, obesity, smoking and deficiencies of folate and vitamin B_{12} (Prince et al. 2007a). All these factors are associated with poor lifestyle and nutritional deficiencies, with tobacco use being greater in LMICs (Prince 2010).

Conclusions and recommendations for mental health promotion in LMICs

The importance of mental health promotion in LMICs is highlighted by the social determinants of mental ill health across the lifespan, most of which are poverty related and malleable. Poor mental health results from the interplay of multiple risk influences and a paucity of protective influences at the different ecological levels in the context of developmental vulnerabilities. An ecological and developmental approach to mental health promotion that takes into account these multiple determinants is thus recommended.

Distal policy-level interventions to reduce exposure to the many social and economic determinants of poor mental in LMICs are crucial. Proximal- and individual-level interventions to promote resilience in the context of risk are, however, equally important. These carry the potential to break the cycle of poverty and mental ill health and contribute to the development of the human capital asset base of LMICs, central to broader socioeconomic development of these countries (Lund et al. 2011).

In the face of the greater burden of life-threatening communicable diseases, it is not surprising that mental health services, and especially mental health promotion, is placed on the backburner in the allocation of scarce resources in LMICs. To increase the public health priority of mental health promotion, advocacy efforts are needed to enlighten governments, policy makers and donor agencies on the role that mental health promotion can play in the promotion of health in general, and the prevention of communicable and non-communicable disease as discussed in the section on the importance of mental health promotion. For example, mental disorders are associated with cardiovascular disease risk factors, such as smoking as well as type 2 diabetes; as well as increased risk for high-risk sexual behaviour associated with HIV infection (Prince et al. 2007b). In addition, the case needs to be made for how mental health promotion can strengthen human and broader socioeconomic development in LMICs. As the social and economic determinants of mental health demand a multisectoral response, these advocacy endeavours need to reach beyond the health sector to harness the collaboration of other sectors.

Existing evidence on poverty-related social determinants of mental ill health provide a good starting point for such efforts. Evidence of the longer-term impact of mental health promotion activities on improving human development and socioeconomic outcomes of beneficiaries and participants in LMICs is, however, sparse. There is, thus, an urgent need for studies demonstrating the overall health and economic benefits of mental health promotion interventions across the lifespan.

In the context of scarce resources, task shifting is recommended as a strategy for the delivery of mental health promotion interventions in LMICs. Given the intersectoral nature of mental health promotion, there are many possible human resources that could be harnessed to this end, including early childhood development workers, teachers, youth workers, health workers, social welfare workers, community development and last but not least, community members themselves. There is emerging evidence from LMICs that community members can be successfully trained to deliver proximal mental health promotion interventions (Bell et al. 2008; Cooper et al. 2009). Harnessing community resources in this way is also important to increase the control of community members over their mental health and advance the principle of empowerment, a central tenet of the practice of health promotion.

Mini toolkit

Tips for effective practice

- Make the case for mental health promotion in LMICs with policy makers and NGOs as an effective way of preventing mental disorders in these countries.
- Seek to address the social determinants of mental ill health, arising from poverty, conflict and gender for example, alongside individual promotion and prevention.
- Adopt a lifespan developmental approach for mental health promotion.
- Ensure that interventions in LMICs are culturally relevant and are shaped by local communities to ensure better fit with local needs and circumstances.

- Ensure sustainability of programmes through building the capacity of local practitioners and NGOS to develop public mental health work.
- Seek to build evidence of the effectiveness of mental health promotion interventions through using low-cost evaluation measures.

Case study

A number of case studies have been used within this chapter to illustrate specific contexts. In addition, a range of further examples and resources can be found at WHO 'QualityRights' project that has recently been launched at www.who.int/mental_health/policy/quality_rights.

Undertaking research and evaluation

- Be aware of the motivation of potential research funders and guard against potentially exploitative research. Research and evaluation should be ethical and invest in local research capacity.
- Ensure that research and evaluation does not ignore poverty and inequalities and consider how to measure the impact of a programme on mental health equity as well as mental health gain.
- Develop research methodology that acknowledges the tension that exists between universal and culturally relativist views of mental health and illness.

Reflection points and questions

- Are mental health promotion efforts at the individual and proximal levels justifiable given evidence on the social determinants of mental ill health that require distal-level interventions?
- How can we raise the public-health priority of mental health promotion in LMICs given the need to address the existing treatment gaps for mental disorders in these countries?
- How can we best strive to ensure that interventions are both culturally congruent and sustainable in LMICs?
- What are some of the epistemological challenges in providing evidence of the effectiveness of mental health promotion interventions?
- Discuss the difference between moderation and mediation in mental health promotion giving examples.
- Discuss why an ecological-systemic and lifespan-developmental approach is an important conceptual framework for mental health promotion.
- Discuss key mental health promotion interventions at each developmental phase.

Further reading and resources

Barry, M.M. and Jenkins, R. (2007) *Implementing Mental Health Promotion.* Oxford: Churchill Livingstone Elsevier.

Petersen, I., Bhana, A., Flisher, A.J., Swartz, L. and Richter, L. (eds) (2010) *Promoting Mental Health in Scarce-Resource Contexts. Emerging Evidence and Practice.* Cape Town: HSRC Press.

World Health Organization (1986) *Ottawa Charter for Health Promotion.* Ottawa: WHO.

World Health Organization (2001) *Mental Health: New Understanding, New Hope.* Geneva: WHO.

World Health Organization (2001) *Strengthening Mental Health Promotion (Fact sheet 220).* Geneva: WHO.

World Health Organization (2002) *Prevention and Promotion in Mental Health*. Geneva: WHO.
World Health Organization (2004) *Prevention of Mental Disorders*. Geneva: WHO.
World Health Organization (2005) *Promoting Mental Health. Concepts, Emerging Evidence, Practice*. Geneva: WHO.

4

Defining and measuring mental health and wellbeing

Sarah Stewart-Brown

The nature of wellbeing

> We must practise the things which produce happiness since if that is present we have everything and if it is absent we do everything in order to have it (Epicurus).

Wellbeing and its determinants are issues on which everyone has the right to a view and social scientists have been gathering information about those views for some time. Wellbeing has of course been studied and written about throughout the ages by philosophers. During the last half century it has become of interest to psychologists, especially those with an interest in public health approaches (Jahoda 1958; Albee 1982). Since then, psychologists have investigated the personal characteristics that tend to be associated with wellbeing and started to develop and evaluate programmes to improve wellbeing at the individual level (Linley and Joseph 2004). Public health and health promotion practitioners have researched and developed ways to improve mental wellbeing at population level (Tudor 1996). There is some overlap between the views of these different groups but also some differences. The most important area of agreement is that wellbeing is more than the absence of 'ill-being' or disease. Another area of agreement is that wellbeing is holistic, covering mental, social and physical components. Unlike discussion about disease where the physical predominates, in discussion about wellbeing, it is the mental, emotional and psychological aspects on which discussion focuses. So, for example, in social science circles, wellbeing is often taken to be synonymous with happiness or satisfaction with life (Office for National Statistics (ONS) 2011a) and in health circles, wellbeing may be referred to as positive mental health (WHO 2004a). Finally, all are agreed that good relationships with others are a fundamental aspect of wellbeing, but there is some disagreement in terms of which relationships should be taken into account. So while all agree that social support is important for wellbeing, intimate or family relationships are often left out of the picture and societal relationships, for example,' trust in government', are included by some and not others.

The nature of wellbeing has come into focus in the UK recently as the current Prime Minister, David Cameron, has proposed that wellbeing should be monitored and the progress of government and society measured on the basis of changes in wellbeing as well as more traditional economic indicators like gross domestic product. The English ONS has been asked to identify robust measures of wellbeing so there has been a flurry of interest and research on the topic and different perspectives are being debated. The case for promoting wellbeing alongside disease prevention is made in current public health policy documents in the UK (Scottish Government 2009; Department of Health 2010a; Department of Health 2011a) and further afield in Canada, Australia and New Zealand. The need for robust measures has been clearly identified in the policy context as well as elsewhere (Stewart-Brown 2002). It is important that measures really do reflect wellbeing otherwise governments, commissioners of services and practitioners will be misled. But it is also important that measures are practical, that the data on which they are based are simple and quick to gather, and that they are statistically robust. It may be that one measure does not suit all circumstances and that a variety is needed.

Views of different disciplines

Philosophers

Aristotle claimed that happiness is the only goal 'we always choose for its own sake and never as a means to something else' (cited in Velasquez 2009: 120). He and Epicurus, and many other philosophers since, have written about the characteristics that humans should cultivate to live a life in which happiness was maximized. The terms hedonic and eudaimonic wellbeing, still in use today (Ryan and Deci 2001), stem from the writings of these Greek philosophers. Hedonic wellbeing is the experience of happiness, also referred to as subjective wellbeing, or affective wellbeing. It is a feeling; a state of mind that comes and goes and is often determined by circumstances beyond the control of the individual. Both hallucinogenic drugs and alcohol can offer a short cut to hedonic wellbeing, but often at the expense of longer-term wellbeing. It is also possible to find a measure of personal happiness at the expense of others – through getting the better of them in some way. Eudaimonic wellbeing is achieved through the cultivation of character traits and behaviours that are believed to maximize happiness, including the components of Aristotle's good life. The latter have found their way into the thinking of modern psychologists where they are presented as psychological wellbeing (Ryff 1989; Ryff and Keyes 1995). They include self-acceptance, environmental mastery or agency, autonomy, purpose in life, personal growth and positive relations with others, and entail engagement with the existential challenges of life (Keyes et al. 2002).

Eastern philosophers have also written much about happiness and how it is attained (Ricard 2003). Buddhist philosophy goes beyond identifying the necessary characteristics and prescribes a path for developing happiness (Ekman et al. 2005). Regular meditation can train the mind to focus on the positive. Acceptance and compassion for self and other enables the mastery of fear, aggression, envy and pride, which cause so many problems in relationships. This path is one that has delivered some extraordinarily contented, resilient individuals and is now being westernized by psychologists and taught to patients and the public as 'mindfulness'. The evidence base on mindfulness and its capacity to promote wellbeing is growing (Kabat-Zim 2003; Grossman et al. 2004; Ludwig and Kabat-Zim 2008) and the idea of regular exercise of the mind is entirely consistent with neuroscientific principles of brain development, which we now know to be a largely use it or lose it affair.

Psychologists

Positive psychologists have developed many important concepts relevant to wellbeing in addition to the psychological wellbeing scales mentioned above. These encourage a focus on the positive rather than on pathological states, and they have provided the backdrop for the current English government's 'Five Ways to Wellbeing' campaign, urging people to: connect, be active, take notice, keep learning and give.

Positive psychologists have also introduced the concept of 'flourishing' (Keyes 2002) conceived as composite of hedonic wellbeing, positive psychological functioning and social wellbeing. In this model, the latter comprises social acceptance, social actualization, social contribution, social coherence and social integration. Investigating the concept of flourishing led Keyes to agree with earlier writers (Tudor 1996) that mental wellbeing and mental illness were not necessarily two opposite ends of a single continuum. Keyes provided evidence that people could languish without mental illness and flourish with it (Keyes 2002). This idea has been influential and popular among those interested in recovery from mental illness, because a single continuum concept seems to deny those with a diagnosis of mental illness the possibility of enjoying wellbeing at any stage in their lives (Weich et al. 2011).

Other key concepts from positive psychologists are those of flow (Csikszentmihalyi and Csikszentmihalyi 1988), signature strengths (Seligman 2002) and emotional intelligence (Salovey and Sluyter 1997). Flow is the focused, absorbed mental state achieved by artists, athletes and others in which a sense of time is lost; a state which has parallels with the meditative state and leads to a sense of fulfilment and contentment. Signature strengths are the positive character traits that enable happiness. Seligman proposes that people identify and find ways of employing their signature strengths in their day-to-day lives. Emotional intelligence and the closely related concept of emotional literacy are the key skills for positive relationship with others. Although they can be learnt throughout life, most validated programmes are based in schools (Greenberg et al. 1995). Although there is complete consensus that good relationships with others are a part of mental wellbeing, the measurement of emotional literacy seems, surprisingly, to have only been raised as relevant for wellbeing in the context of children.

Social scientists

The foregoing discussion suggests that the boundaries between the approaches and beliefs of the different disciplines are far from rigid and there is evidence of them being crossed by many individuals. Nevertheless, they retain an explanatory value. On the whole, social scientists have investigated wellbeing using simple measures of life satisfaction and happiness (Diener et al. 1985). They have endeavoured to find out which of a variety of social circumstances and structures give rise to the greatest levels of subjective wellbeing. Theirs is the simplest, but least sophisticated approach to measurement. Their underlying belief system – that society rather than individuals themselves hold all the trump cards when it comes to determining wellbeing – contrasts with that of the psychologists and indeed many philosophers. As a generality, they also believe that the individual's subjective view of their happiness is more reliable than that of the experts who have reflected, observed, studied and experimented. For much of modern history, social scientists have espoused the belief that income was the most important determinant of individual's wellbeing and this belief system has profoundly influenced Western governments. The report from the Stiglitz commission (Stiglitz et al. 2009), showing the lack of relationship between income and wellbeing has played a key role in stimulating the recent UK government level interest in wellbeing and its measurement.

Views of the public and areas of debate

During the recent debate on the nature of wellbeing, organized by the ONS (2011a), members of the general public were asked to rank determinants of wellbeing in order of importance and they came up with the following: health, good connections with friends and family, job satisfaction, economic security and present and future conditions of the environment. Many respondents added to the list and the most frequent contributions were: availability of green spaces, work–life balance, cultural and creative activities, fairness and equality, community spirit, trustworthy government and quality of government provided services. These findings were echoed in a similar exercises carried out by Department for Environment, Food and Rural Affairs (DEFRA 2011) and by the Organization for Economic and Cooperative Development (OECD 2011a). Such surveys do not give a picture of what the public think wellbeing is and tend to invite external rather than internal solutions to wellbeing. In the social scientists' view of determinants, community spirit and good connections with family and friends seem to be presented as something that it is the responsibility of others to provide. The psychologists and philosophers, in contrast, would tend to view this as something individuals can influence for themselves through the way they treat others and the effort they put into cultivating community spirit in their localities. Social scientists tend to go for societal solutions that are popular because effortless to recipients. The solutions of psychologists may seem less attractive in the short term because they involve personal effort but they have the benefit of empowering people and giving them skills to enable their happiness that are not dependent on external circumstances.

The New Economics Foundation presents an exception to this classification with their National Accounts of Wellbeing initiative (nef 2009). Here personal wellbeing is presented as a composite of eudaimonic and hedonic wellbeing (Figure 4.1). This schema explicitly includes resilience, which is perhaps the most widely recognized facet of mental wellbeing in the health world. The WHO's definition of positive mental health includes the ability to 'cope with the normal stresses of life' (WHO 2004a: 12) and English policy's as 'feeling safe and able to cope'

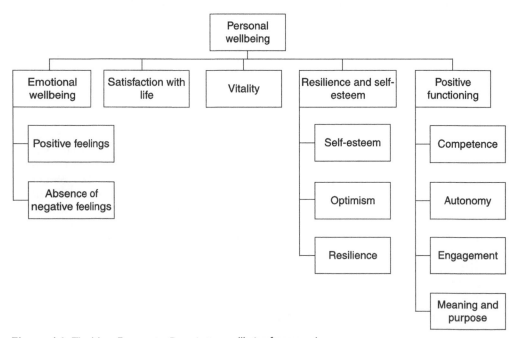

Figure 4.1 The New Economics Foundation wellbeing framework.

Source: Michaelson, J. et al. (2009) *National Accounts of Well-being: Bringing Real Wealth onto the Balance Sheet.* London: nef (see www.nationalaccountsofwellbeing.org)

(Department of Health 2010b: 12). In nef's schema social wellbeing is presented separately as supportive relationships, trust and belonging.

Measurement scales

Box 4.1 lists key measurement scales from the different disciplines and further instruments are available from Psychtests (http://corporate.psychtests.com).

Box 4.1 Wellbeing scales

Social science

- Single-item happiness scales
- Single-item life-satisfaction scales
- Multiple-domain life-satisfaction scales

Psychology

- Positive and Negative Affect Schedule (PANAS)
- Psychological Well-being Scales
- Flourishing/Languishing Scale
- Flourishing Scale
- Emotional Intelligence Scale

General

- Warwick-Edinburgh Mental Well-being Scale (WEMWBS)
- WHO-5 Well-Being Index
- General Health Questionnaire (GHQ-12)

Differences between these measurement scales lie not just in the implicit understanding of wellbeing as hedonic or eudaimonic, but also in their length, the number of scale scores that are derived from the responses and their comprehensibility. Thus, scales range from single questions (How happy are you these days?) to the 54 items of the Psychological Well-being Scales (Ryff and Keyes 1995). Some scales can be used to derive a single score; Warwick-Edinburgh Mental Well-being Scale (WEMWBS, Tennant et al. 2007a), Flourishing/Languishing Scale (Keyes 2002), Flourishing Scale (Deiner et al. 2009), WHO-5 Well-Being Index (Bech 2004), multiple-domain Life Satisfaction (Diener 1984); some two scores such as the Positive and Negative Affect Schedule (PANAS, Watson et al. 1988) and some several scores such as Psychological Well-being (Ryff and Keyes 1995). They also vary in comprehensibility of the items and the sophistication of the concepts they represent. A further widely available measure, the General Health Questionnaire (GHQ-12, see Goldberg and Williams 1988) was developed to identify common mental disorders, yet is often used as an indicator of mental wellbeing in the general population. In this situation scores are simply reversed to measure wellbeing (Hu et al. 2007).

This list does not include some notable wellbeing indicators being proposed today, for example that of the OECD (2011a) or United Nations Children's Fund (UNICEF 2007). These are scales that were developed very much in the social science tradition, where the focus is on societal determinants of wellbeing. The latter have the advantage that they can be derived from data available in individual countries and that the data are mainly based on objective measures. They have the disadvantage of being proxy measures of wellbeing. Although all the determinants are supported by a robust evidence base, the extent to which they actually determine wellbeing (the population attributable risk in public health terms) is very variable and usually small. Because outcome measures dictate which interventions, projects and programmes are deemed to be effective, proxy measures have the potential to be profoundly misleading.

Measurement issues

Some measurement issues are mentioned above, for example, the extent to which measures are based on single simple questions with strong face validity and low respondent burden versus the extent to which they represent a more sophisticated view of wellbeing. Another issue mentioned above but worthy of repetition is the issue of whether mental health can be represented as a single continuum from mental wellbeing to mental illness. Single factor scales such as WEMWBS or the GHQ-12 imply a single spectrum. The fact that these two scales are very highly correlated (Tennant et al. 2007a) when the GHQ-12 is scored continuously as opposed to the normal dichotomous scoring suggest that it is not unreasonable to take this view. The main evidence to the contrary is based on correlation with diagnosis of mental illness. The latter includes a wide spectrum of disability from the severely disabled to those who have overcome the enormous obstacles this type of illness poses and effectively recovered from the illness, albeit taking small doses of maintenance drugs. One could argue that the problem here is the medical label, which for psychotic illness is a life-long affair, not the assessment of wellbeing.

A further issue, touched on above, is the extent to which measures depend on subjective reporting or objective facts. The latter are usually preferred, but not available for large-scale surveys. Wellbeing can be observed and rated objectively but measurement is costly. The objective measures of wellbeing that appear in the literature are almost invariably measures of potential or actual determinants of wellbeing.

Finally, the scales vary in the extent to which they represent a balance between the positive and the negative (Psychological Well-being Scales, PANAS, Emotional Intelligence Scale) or focus entirely on the positive (WEMWBS, Flourishing/Languishing Scale, Flourishing Scale, WHO-5). Older scales like the GHQ-12 comprise items covering similar topics, but they are distinguished by their focus on the negative. Balanced scales are considered by some to be ideal because they are thought to be least likely to be subject to block responding (ticking a single level in a Lickert scale for all items). On the other hand, wholly positive measures are very popular with those undertaking mental health promotion initiatives. Scales like WEMWBS implicitly present a positive goal to participants conveying the belief that practitioners or providers hope to enable participants to develop greater wellbeing. In contrast negatively oriented scales like the GHQ-12 implicitly convey the message that practitioners are only really interested in participants if they are mentally ill and aim only to prevent more illness. The difference is subtle but can make an impact on the acceptability of the project.

Mini toolkit

Tips for effective practice
- Views on the determinants of mental health and wellbeing differ with some favouring models based on personal development and some on external conditions. Both models are

likely to be pertinent and their effects interactive. Practitioners should discuss their beliefs about the relationship between structure and agency in determining wellbeing as this should shape the measures you employ.

• Consider triangulating different measures of wellbeing at the individual, community and structural level to provide a comprehensive picture of population mental health.

Case study: The Warwick-Edinburgh Mental Well-Being Scale (WEMWBS)

The WEMWBS is a prototype measure of mental wellbeing that is proving very popular in the UK and further afield. It was developed (Tennant et al. 2007a) using funding provided by the Scottish Government as part of their new mental health strategy. The central tenet of development was that the instrument would focus on positive aspects of mental health identified in the literature. It therefore combines both eudaimonic and hedonic components. It is also short, readily understood and recognized as an instrument of mental wellbeing by the general public. The completed instrument includes 14 items, all of which are positively worded; it has five levels of response to be assessed over a two-week period, from none of the time to all of the time (see Figure 4.2).

The original validation of WEMWBS was undertaken in a large representative population in Scotland, with a group of students at Scottish and English universities and with focus groups in both countries (Tennant et al. 2007a, 2007b). Although the student sample, in particular, and Scottish and English populations more generally, are multicultural, White British responses were predominant in the validation and the youngest contributors were 16 years old. Further validation studies have been undertaken with English-speaking minority ethnic groups living in the UK, Italians in Italy, Setswana-speaking populations in South Africa (Stewart-Brown 2013) and 13- to 15-year-olds in UK schools (Clarke et al. 2011). In all these settings WEMWBS has proved valid, suggesting that it is robust to translation and across cultures, down to age 13 years. Qualitative evaluation suggests that some items were less readily grasped than others; one of these was the item 'I feel optimistic about the future'. Norms for another item 'I've been able to make up my own mind about things' were different in Pakistani communities to the general population for cultural reasons, and one item 'I've been interested in other people' was interpreted by some young people as being about romantic attraction. These comments offer thought for further development of WEMWBS when the time is right, but do not invalidate its use at present.

A Rasch model analysis (Stewart-Brown et al. 2009) has provided information on the measurement properties of WEMWBS. With Rasch model compatibility, a scale score difference of 5–10 can be assumed to be the same as 20–25. The 14-item WEMWBS was not compatible with the model but a shortened version comprising seven items (SWEMWBS) was. The SWEMWBS has the advantage of low-respondent burden, so it is valued in large surveys, but because it has fewer items it presents a more limited view of wellbeing to study participants. Fewer items also mean less chance of demonstrating change. In the latter regard, the full 14-item scale is responsive to change both at the group level and at the level of the individual. Projects as diverse as parenting programmes, complementary and alternative medicine projects for carers of people with mental illness and psychiatric day hospital attendance produced significant changes in WEMWBS score (Maheswaran et al. in press) with relatively modest samples.

Practitioners in the UK say that they used to feel very ambivalent about evaluating their mental health promoting projects with existing scales, whose items focus on, for example, feeling 'down in the dumps'. However, WEMWBS, in contrast, seems to work very well in this context. Practitioners say that it is as though the instrument proclaims the purpose of

Below are some statements about feelings and thoughts.

Please tick the box that best describes your experience of each over the last 2 weeks STATEMENTS	None of the time	Rarely	Some of the time	Often	All of the time
I've been feeling optimistic about the future	1	2	3	4	5
I've been feeling useful	1	2	3	4	5
I've been feeling relaxed	1	2	3	4	5
I've been feeling interested in other people	1	2	3	4	5
I've had energy to spare	1	2	3	4	5
I've been dealing with problems well	1	2	3	4	5
I've been thinking clearly	1	2	3	4	5
I've been feeling good about myself	1	2	3	4	5
I've been feeling close to other people	1	2	3	4	5
I've been feeling confident	1	2	3	4	5
I've been able to make up my own mind about things	1	2	3	4	5
I've been feeling loved	1	2	3	4	5
I've been interested in new things	1	2	3	4	5
I've been feeling cheerful	1	2	3	4	5

Figure 4.2 The Warwick-Edinburgh Mental Well-Being Scale (WEMWBS). ©NHS Health Scotland, University of Warwick, University of Edinburgh, 2006, all rights reserved.

their projects in terms of 'this is what we want for you'. Because focusing on the positive changes the nature of interventions, evaluation with WEMWBS has, at some level, become a mental health promoting intervention in its own right. In addition, WEMWBS has been incorporated into key national health surveys in Scotland and England as well as into a host of other large surveys and cohort studies. In Scotland, a reduction in WEWMBS score is now one of seven health targets for the Scottish Government.

The development of WEMWBS represents an initiative that is of its time. It is supporting the development of public health in the UK and also in other settings by countering the argument that mental wellbeing cannot be measured and by enabling robust evaluation of projects. As concepts of mental wellbeing get further debated and investigated and as we develop a wider repertoire of approaches to improving mental wellbeing involving for example positive psychology approaches, mindfulness, emotional literacy, community development and arts for health projects, it is likely that WEMWBS will be superseded by other instruments, but at present it is serving a useful purpose in many different respects.

Reflection points and questions

* Does the selection of a measure of mental wellbeing imply a belief about the determinants of wellbeing and the best approaches to improving wellbeing?
* In what circumstances is it appropriate to adopt a single-item measure of wellbeing and what circumstances warrant more sophisticated measures?
* Should we measure wellbeing or its determinants and why?

Further reading and resources

* Ryan, R.M. and Deci, E.L. (2001) On happiness and human potentials: a review of research on hedonic and eudaimonic wellbeing, *Annual Review of Psychology*, 52: 141–166.
* Reports by the Commission on Measurement of Economic Performance and Social Progress. Available at http://www.stiglitz-sen-fitoussi.fr/en/documents.htm (accessed 22 August 2012).
* Ricard, M. (2003) *Happiness: A Guide to Life's Most Important Skill*. New York: Little, Brown and Company.
* New Economics Foundation interactive website at www.nationalaccountsofwellbeing. org/ (accessed 22 August 2012).
* Psychtests directory at http://corporate.psychtests.com/ (accessed 22 August 2012).

Part 2
Preventing mental health problems

5 Inequality: an underacknowledged source of mental illness and distress

Kate E Pickett and Richard G Wilkinson

Summary

Greater income inequality is associated with higher prevalence of mental illness and drug misuse in rich societies. There are threefold differences in the proportion of the population suffering from mental illness between more and less equal countries. This relationship is most likely mediated by the impact of inequality on the quality of social relationships and the scale of status differentiation in different societies.

Introduction

Studies have shown that physical health is better, levels of trust higher and violence lower in societies where income is more equally distributed (Wilkinson and Pickett 2006). When income differences are measured at the level of whole nations or very large regions, such as the American states, the evidence for a negative effect of inequality on health is highly consistent, and multilevel studies have shown that this impact is not confounded by individual income or socioeconomic status or the curvilinear relationship between income and inequality (Wolfson et al. 1999; Subramanian and Kawachi 2004; Wilkinson and Pickett 2006; Kondo et al. 2009). Studies that have examined income inequality within smaller regions and neighbourhoods provide much less consistent evidence. For example, a study of income inequality in British regions found an increased risk in scores on the GHQ for rich people, but not for poor people (Weich et al. 2001). We believe that measuring income inequality within sub-national or sub-state areas is inappropriate; deprived areas have poorer health, not because of inequalities within them, but because they are poor relative to the wider society. It seems to be the degree of social stratification across the whole society that matters for population health, which also means that ecological studies are the most appropriate study design in this field of research.

We have recently shown that other health and social problems, including mental illness, are also more common in more unequal societies (Wilkinson and Pickett 2007, 2009a, 2010). These relationships reflect human sensitivity to social relations and to the impact of income inequality on the scale of social hierarchy and status competition in a society.

The burden of mental health problems in the UK today is very high. For example, estimates suggest that one million British children – one in ten between the ages of 5 and 16 – are mentally ill and that in any secondary school with 1000 students, 50 will have severe depression, 100 will be distressed, between 10 and 20 will have obsessive–compulsive disorder and between 5 and 10 girls will have an eating disorder (Donnellan 2004). Among UK adults, in a national survey conducted in 2000, 23 per cent of adults had a mental illness in the previous 12 months, and 4 per cent of adults had had more than one disorder in the previous year (ONS 2001). In the USA, one in four adults have been mentally ill in the past year and almost a quarter of these episodes were severe; over their lifetime more than half of US adults will experience mental illness.

Income inequality and rates of mental illness

But are such levels of mental illness an inevitable consequence of modern life in high-income societies? Not at all. Rates of mental illness vary substantially between rich societies. Comparable data on the prevalence of mental illness – free from cultural differences in reporting, diagnosis, categorization and treatment have only recently become available. In 1998, WHO established the World Mental Health Survey Consortium to estimate the prevalence of mental illness in different countries, the severity of illness and patterns of treatment. Although their methods do not entirely overcome worries about cultural differences in interpreting and responding to such questions, at least the same diagnostic interviews are used in each country.

We used these data as part of our investigation into the impact of income inequality on health and social problems; we examined the prevalence of mental illness in the WHO surveys from Belgium, France, Germany, Italy, Japan, The Netherlands, New Zealand, Spain and the USA (Demyttenaere et al. 2004; Wells et al. 2006), and from three national surveys using similar methodology from Australia (Australian Bureau of Statistics 2003), Canada (WHO 2000) and the UK (ONS 2001). Figure 5.1 shows the association in rich countries between income inequality and the proportion of adults who have been mentally ill in the 12 months prior to being interviewed. This is a strong relationship ($r=0.73$, $P<0.01$), and clearly a much higher percentage of the population have a mental illness in more unequal countries; only Italy is somewhat of an outlier, with lower levels of mental illness than we might expect on the basis of its level of income inequality. Inequality is associated with threefold differences in prevalence: in Germany, Italy, Japan and Spain, fewer than one in ten people have been mentally ill within the past year; in Australia, Canada, New Zealand and the UK it is more than one in five people, and in the USA more than one in four.

Among the nine countries with data from WHO surveys, we can also examine subtypes of mental illness, specifically, anxiety disorders, mood disorders, impulse–control disorders and addictions, as well as a measure of severe mental illness. Anxiety disorders, impulse–control disorders and severe illness are all strongly correlated with inequality, mood disorders less so. Anxiety disorders represent the largest subgroup in all these countries, and the percentage of all mental illnesses that are anxiety disorders is itself significantly higher in more unequal countries.

As a separate test of the hypothesis that greater income inequality leads to an increase in the prevalence of mental illness, we repeated our analysis within the 50 states of the USA. State-specific estimates of mental illness are collected by the United States Behavioural Risk Factor Surveillance Study (Zahran et al. 2005). We found that state-level income inequality is significantly associated with mental illness in adult women and with the percentage of children in

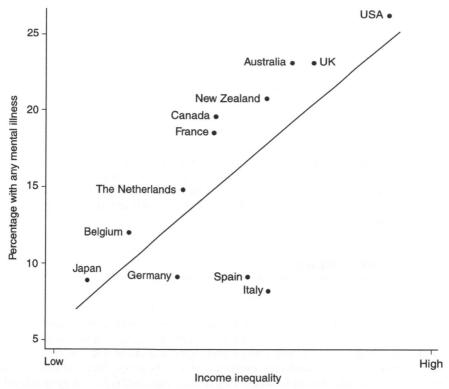

Figure 5.1 More people have mental illnesses in more unequal countries.

each state with 'moderate or severe difficulties in the area of emotions, concentration, behaviour, or getting along with others' (Child and Adolescent Health Measurement Initiative (CAHMI) 2006: para. 3). However, we found no association for adult men. This may be related to gender differences in willingness to report mental illness in the USA, as these data are self-reported mental illness rather than being derived from diagnostic interviews. Among other US-based studies none have used diagnostic interviewers, however, studies have shown that state-level (Fiscella and Franks 2000) and county-level (Kahn et al. 2000) income inequality are associated with a significant increased risk of reporting depressive symptoms, and state-level inequality is associated with self-reported mental health (Shi et al. 2002). Only one study found no effect for depressive symptoms (Henderson et al. 2004).

Why do more people tend to have mental health problems in more unequal places? Psychologist Oliver James uses an analogy with infectious disease to explain the link. What James terms the 'affluenza' virus is a 'set of values which increase our vulnerability to emotional distress', and he argues that these values are more common in affluent societies (James 2007: vii). They entail placing a high value on acquiring money and possessions, looking good in the eyes of others and wanting to be famous. He goes on to argue that these values increase the risk of depression, anxiety, substance misuse and personality disorder. Philosopher Alain de Botton claims that our anxiety about our social status is 'a worry so pernicious as to be capable of ruining extended stretches of our lives' (de Botton 2004: 3–4). When we fail to maintain our position in the social hierarchy we are 'condemned to consider the successful with bitterness and ourselves with shame' (de Botton 2004: 5). Economist Robert Frank calls the same phenomenon 'luxury fever' (Frank 1999). As inequality increases and the super rich at the top spend more and more on luxury goods, the desire for such things cascades down the income scale and the rest of us struggle to compete and keep up. Advertisers play on this, making us dissatisfied with what we have, and encouraging invidious social comparisons – more unequal societies spend more in advertising (Wilkinson and Pickett 2010). Economist Richard Layard describes us as having an 'addiction to income' – the more we have, the more we feel we need and the more time we spend on striving for material wealth and possessions, at the expense of our family life, relationships and quality of life (Layard 2005: 49).

Although not all these authors make the link specifically with income inequality, it is not surprising that the tendencies they describe are stronger in more unequal societies. Our impression is that greater inequality increases status competition and status insecurity. Internationally and among the 50 states of the USA, income inequality is strongly related to low levels of trust, to weaker community life and to increased violence. Mental health is profoundly influenced by the quality and sufficiency of social relationships and all these measures suggest that both are harmed by inequality.

Inequality and drug misuse

We have also found that the use of illegal drugs, such as cocaine, marijuana and heroin, is more common in more unequal societies. The United Nations (UN) Office on Drugs and Crime publishes a World Drug report (UN Office on Drugs and Crime 2007), which contains separate data on the use of opiates, cocaine, cannabis, ecstasy and amphetamines. Combining these into a single index (equally weighted, using z-scores), we found a strong tendency for drug use to be more common in more unequal countries ($r=0.63$, $P<0.01$). Within the 50 American states, there is also a tendency for addiction to illegal drugs and deaths from drug overdose to be higher in the more unequal states (Center for Disease Control and Prevention 2007).

Although we must be cautious in extrapolating to humans, animal studies show that low social status profoundly affects neurological systems. Researchers at Wake Forest School of Medicine housed 20 macaque monkeys in individual cages (Morgan et al. 2002). They next housed the animals in groups of four and observed the social hierarchies that developed in each group, noting which animals were dominant and which subordinate. They scanned the monkeys' brains before and after they were put into groups. Next, they taught the monkeys that they could administer cocaine to themselves by pressing a lever – they could take as much or as little as they liked. Monkeys that had become dominant had higher levels of dopamine activity than they had exhibited before becoming dominant, whereas monkeys that became subordinate when housed in groups showed no changes in dopamine, and the dominant monkeys took significantly less cocaine than the subordinate monkeys. The subordinate monkeys medicated themselves against the impact of their low social status. This kind of experimental animal evidence adds plausibility to our inference that inequality is causally related to mental illness.

As well as trust, social capital, violence, mental illness and drug misuse, income inequality is also linked to physical morbidity and mortality, to low social mobility and poor educational achievement, to bullying in schools, and rates of imprisonment, teenage births and the status of women in society. As inequality grows, so do the social distances and distinctions between us, and so does the potential for the pain of low social status, stigma and shame (Friedli 2009). To a great extent, we see ourselves through each other's eyes and, in more unequal societies more of us find ourselves wanting in those reflections.

But what are the clinical and policy implications of our findings? The most recent review of health inequalities in England (the Marmot Review) calls attention to the need to tackle the individual causes of poor health across the life-course, and acknowledges the social gradient in health, whereby even the health of those close to the top of society is worse than those at the very top (Marmot 2010). But the Marmot Review, although it calls for a minimum income for healthy living, fails to deal with the real implications of research on income inequality and health and social problems – we have to constrain runaway salaries and the bonus culture as well as raising the incomes of the poorest.

Implications

The clinical implications of our results are relatively straightforward. If people suffer mental distress as a consequence of low social status, stigma and shame, then their treatment must emphasize their human worth and be conducted within a respectful relationship. The policy implications are more diverse and numerous, but fall into two camps. To make the UK a more equal and consequently a healthier and happier society, we must redistribute income through taxes and benefits, find ways to reduce income differences in market incomes before taxes, or both. Research suggests that the key to the latter strategy is strong trade unions. But ways of reducing income differences before taxes might also include employee representation on corporate remuneration boards, greater transparency in salary ratios in both the public and private sector, and all forms of institutional democracy – cooperatives, mutual societies, employee-owned companies, etc. If we want to commit the UK to as rapid a reversal of inequality as the massive rise experienced during the 1980s, then we need to encourage all mechanisms that help to reduce income differences. As professionals dedicated to improving the health of the population, our role in calling for greater equality is as important in the twenty-first century as the efforts of the great public health reformers of the Victorian era who called for improvements in sanitation, housing, nutrition and working conditions.

To end on an optimistic note, it is worth remembering that the UK has not always been among the most unequal of the rich, market democracies. Our current inequality, and our unacceptably high prevalence of mental and physical illness, as well as other health and social problems, is not a fixed characteristic of British culture – we used to be more equal, and we could be so again.

Further reading and resources

- The Equality Trust: www.equalitytrust.org.uk
- Public Health and Social Justice: http://phsj.org
- UCL Institute of Health Equity: www.instituteofhealthequity.org

Previously published by The Royal College of Psychiatrists. Kate E. Pickett and Richard G. Wilkinson (2010) Inequality: an underacknowledged source of mental illness and distress. *The British Journal of Psychiatry*, 197: 426-428. © The Royal College of Psychiatrists.

6 Mental health literacy

Nicola J Reavley and Anthony F Jorm

Introduction

In recent decades, significant resources have been invested in education, screening and treatment facilities to help members of the public prevent, obtain treatment for and manage physical health conditions. Highly visible health education campaigns have focused on the links between sun exposure and skin cancer, the importance of diet and exercise in reducing the risk of cardiovascular disease and the role of safe sex in preventing the transmission of HIV. Many members of the public know the appropriate sources of professional help available for physical health conditions, some of treatments they might receive, and the likely benefits of those treatments. They may also be familiar with available complementary treatments and lifestyle changes they might make. Such knowledge also benefits others around them; someone who has taken a first aid course to learn how to apply cardiopulmonary resuscitation in an emergency may save a life.

This situation can be contrasted with that for mental disorders. Many people do not recognize the signs and symptoms of these disorders, have beliefs about prevention and treatment that diverge from those of health professionals and are not sure how to help someone with a mental disorder. This is surprising in the context of the high prevalence rates of mental disorders. In any one year, between 10 and 19 per cent of people experience a mental disorder, and lifetime prevalence rates vary between 18 and 36 per cent (Kessler et al. 2009). Depression, anxiety and related disorders are among the leading causes of disability worldwide (Kessler et al. 2005a; WHO 2008).

Help-seeking for mental disorders

A common finding across surveys in many countries is that, although mental disorder prevalence rates are high, many people either do not seek or delay seeking help, often for many years.

The WHO's World Health Initiative examined data from 28 developed and developing coun-tries (Wang et al. 2007a). These surveys showed that, even in developed countries, only a minority of people received treatment for mood, anxiety or substance use disorders in the year of disorder onset. For those who eventually received treatment, the median delays ranged from 1 to 14 years for mood disorders, 3 to 30 years for anxiety disorders, and 6 to 18 years for substance use disorders. Even for the more severe disorders, such as psychosis, delays of months are typical (Marshall et al. 2005).

Delays in seeking treatment are important because early intervention improves the prognosis for those with mental disorders. There is convincing evidence that a longer duration of untreated disease is associated with adverse outcomes for psychosis (Marshall et al. 2005), depression (Altamura et al. 2008a), anxiety disorders (Altamura et al. 2008b) and bipolar disorder (Altamura et al. 2010).

A number of factors, both individual and structural, interact to determine when and how people seek help for mental health problems. Individual factors include knowledge and atti-tudes and structural factors include family, community support systems and health system structures.

Mental health literacy

In the mid-1990s, the term *mental health literacy* was coined to focus attention on the low levels of knowledge about mental disorders in the community. It is defined as 'knowledge and beliefs about mental disorders which aid their recognition, management or prevention' (Jorm et al. 1997: 182). Although mental health literacy incorporates knowledge about mental disorders, it goes further in that it places emphasis on the knowledge being linked to the possibility of action to benefit one's own mental health or that of others. Mental health literacy incorporates:

- knowing how to prevent mental disorders;
- recognition of when a disorder is developing to facilitate early help-seeking;
- knowledge of help-seeking options and available treatments;
- knowing effective self-help strategies for milder problems;
- first aid skills to support others who are developing a mental disorder or in a mental health crisis.

For someone with a mental disorder, mental health literacy also incorporates knowledge of how to manage an illness, whereas for a caregiver, it covers knowledge of how to provide effective support to the person with the illness. Such education is often provided by a health profes-sional. In this chapter, the focus is on those aspects of mental health literacy that apply to the community as a whole.

Recognition of developing mental disorders to facilitate early help-seeking

A key factor in determining whether a person receives professional help for a mental health problem is recognition of the problem as a mental disorder (Gulliver et al. 2010). In an Australian study of people being treated for anxiety or mood disorders, the average time between onset of symptoms and help-seeking was 8.2 years (Thompson et al. 2008). Within this period, it took an average of 6.9 years to recognize the problem, and an average of 1.3 years between recognition and help-seeking.

Concern about low levels of mental health literacy has led to the conduct of studies in a number of countries. In such surveys, recognition is commonly assessed by presenting respondents with a case vignette describing a person with a mental disorder and asking them what they think is wrong with the person. Although the ability to give the correct label varies according to the disorder described and the nationality of the respondent, underrecognition is common. Rates of recognition for depression vary between 50 and 86 per cent (Jorm et al. 2005a; Wang et al. 2007a; Dahlberg et al. 2008; Reavley and Jorm 2011a), whereas recognition of other disorders, such as psychosis/schizophrenia or anxiety disorders, tends to be lower (Jorm et al. 2005a; Wright et al. 2005; Pescosolido et al. 2008; Wright and Jorm 2009; Reavley and Jorm 2011a).

Rather than using disorder labels, participants in such surveys often use terms such as 'stress' or 'life problem'. Results of Australian surveys assessing depression literacy suggest that people who use labels other than depression are more likely to believe in the helpfulness of dealing with the problem alone (Jorm et al. 2006a; Wright et al. 2007).

Knowledge of professional help and effective treatments available

Although recognition of a problem as a mental disorder is critical to facilitating help-seeking, it is only the first step as, in order to get effective help, the person also needs to know about the range of professional help and evidence-based treatments available to them. Moreover, people need to believe that the services offered by health professionals can be helpful.

Surveys of public beliefs about professionals and treatments have been carried out in many developed countries (Priest et al. 1996; Jorm 2000; Lauber et al. 2001; Croghan et al. 2003; Magliano et al. 2004; Angermeyer et al. 2005; Jorm et al. 2005a; Reavley and Jorm 2011a). Common findings include the following.

- Most people have positive views of family and friends as a source of help, often ahead of health professionals (Jorm et al. 2000a; Burns and Rapee 2006; Jorm and Wright 2007).
- Many people view psychiatric medications negatively due to concerns that they do not treat the underlying causes and can cause dependence (Pyne et al. 2005).
- Psychological treatments such as counselling are viewed very positively for a wide range of disorders (Jorm et al. 1997; Lauber et al. 2001; Kovess-Masfety et al. 2007; Wang et al. 2007b; Reavley and Jorm 2011a).
- Beliefs about general practitioners (GPs) as a source of help for mental disorders are very positive in most countries, although the nature of the healthcare system and the perceived appropriateness of GPs for mental health treatment have an impact on beliefs.
- A significant minority of the population believes that it is helpful to deal with mental disorders on one's own (ten Have et al. 2009).

Knowledge of effective self-help strategies

Self-help strategies are actions that a person can take to deal with a mental disorder on their own. Such strategies are typically used informally without any professional guidance, although in some cases they may be used with the guidance of a health professional as part of psychological therapy (for example use of a book or website providing CBT). Commonly used informal self-help strategies include the use of alcohol to relax, pain relievers, physical activity, help from family and friends, holidays and time off work (Jorm et al. 2000b). Community surveys indicate that self-help strategies such as taking vitamins, physical activity, reading about the problem, getting out more, following a special diet, and doing courses on relaxation, stress management or yoga tend to be viewed very positively, often more so than professional mental disorder treatments (Reavley and Jorm 2011a). Although some of these strategies, including physical activity, may be helpful, others such as the use of alcohol may contribute to the worsening of symptoms (Jorm et al. 2002). There is also a concern that the use of self-help strategies may be used as an alternative to professional help (Jorm et al. 2000b).

Knowledge and skills to give mental health first aid and support to others

Given the high prevalence of mental disorders in the community, there is a high likelihood of coming into contact with someone with a mental health problem. Friends or family members often recognize that someone is developing a disorder and it is therefore beneficial for members of the public to know how they can assist and support someone in these circumstances. Appropriate help and support may facilitate both recognition and help-seeking and may play a significant role in a person's recovery from a mental disorder. There is evidence that people experiencing a mental disorder are more likely to seek professional help if someone else suggests it (Dew et al. 1991; Cusack et al. 2004). Another way in which people in the social network can assist is to provide ongoing social support. For example, there is evidence that positive social support helps reduce the impact of traumatic life events and that recovery from depression is assisted when family members provide good social support (Keitner et al. 1995; Charuvastra and Cloitre 2008).

Such assistance may be termed *mental health first aid*, which has been defined as the initial help provided by a person's social network when they are developing a mental health problem or are in a mental health crisis (Kitchener and Jorm 2002). Given the limited evidence for the most appropriate strategies to use in providing mental health first aid for a broad range of mental disorders and mental health crisis situations, a number of Delphi studies have been carried out to establish expert consensus using panels of mental health professionals, consumers and caregivers (Kelly et al. 2008a, 2008b; Langlands et al. 2008; Hart et al. 2009; Kelly et al. 2009; Kingston et al. 2009; Kelly et al. 2010). These studies have identified eight common elements to providing good mental health first aid. They include: approaching the person, assessing the situation, assisting with any crisis, listening non-judgementally, offering support, offering information, encouraging the person to get professional help and encouraging other supports (including social supports and self-help strategies).

Several Australian surveys have assessed the mental health first aid knowledge of members of the public. A survey of adults presented a range of case vignettes and asked participants what they would do if this was a person they knew and cared about (Jorm et al. 2005b). The most common responses were to encourage professional help-seeking and to listen to and support the person, which is in accordance with the above expert recommendations. However, significant minorities of individuals in the survey did not mention these responses. Of greatest concern was that, when presented with a scenario of a depressed and suicidal individual, only 15 per cent mentioned assessing the risk of harm, an action that is regarded as highly appropriate by mental health professionals (Jorm et al. 2008).

Knowledge of how to prevent mental disorders

The contrast between public knowledge of physical disorders with that of mental disorders is most striking in the area of prevention. Strategies rated as helpful in a German study included stable friendships, enjoyable leisure activities, family support, thinking positively, disclosing oneself to a confidante, activities that increase self-confidence, meaningful activities, getting enough sleep, abstaining from drugs, doing exercise, and relaxing while listening to music

(Schomerus et al. 2008). However, very little is known about what members of the public do in practice for prevention of mental disorders. Although knowledge about the major modifiable risk factors for mental disorders is limited, there is growing evidence in some areas, including cannabis and psychosis (Moore et al. 2007), parenting strategies and substance misuse (Hayes et al. 2004; Lae and Crano 2009) and the effects of family conflict on children (Kelly 2000).

Mental health literacy in young people

It can be argued that improving mental health literacy in young people is of particular importance due to the fact that mental disorders often have first onset during adolescence or early adulthood, a period of life when knowledge and experience are underdeveloped. In the USA, the median age of onset for anxiety disorders has been reported as 11 years, for mood disorders 30 years, and for substance use disorders 20 years (Kessler et al. 2005b). Similar ages of onset have been found in other countries (Kessler et al. 2007).

A number of aspects of mental health literacy appear to be affected by age. Young people are more likely to be able to correctly identify a mental disorder described in a case vignette as they get older (Wright et al. 2007; Wright and Jorm 2009). Recognition is also associated with better help-seeking and treatment preferences (Wright et al. 2007) and self-labelling as having a disorder may also help health practitioners to recognize the young person's problem (Haller et al. 2009). Attitudes to treatment also appear to improve with age (Gonzalez et al. 2009).

Although young people may need the help of parents or other supportive adults to recognize that what they are experiencing is a mental disorder for which they need to seek appropriate professional help, many adolescents prefer to turn to friends as a source of help if they have a mental health problem (Burns and Rapee 2006; Jorm and Wright 2007). However, many young people do not have the experience and maturity to take on this role or to facilitate professional help-seeking. Furthermore, evidence suggests that many young people supporting peers are often reluctant to approach an adult about their concerns (Dunham 2004; Kelly et al. 2006).

All of these surveys looked at stated intentions to provide assistance in hypothetical situations. Only one study has examined actual mental health first aid actions taken (Yap et al. 2011). Results of a survey of young Australians aged 13–28 years showed that the most common responses towards a friend or family member who had a mental health problem were to listen to the person (reported by 91 per cent), encourage physical activity (69 per cent), bring together friends to cheer the person up (67 per cent) and keep the person busy to keep their mind off problems (66 per cent). Only 58 per cent suggested professional help and only 38 per cent asked about suicidal feelings. Some reported doing potentially unhelpful things like talking to the person firmly about getting their act together (45 per cent), suggesting use of alcohol to forget their troubles (6 per cent) or ignoring the person until they got over it (4 per cent). These and the earlier results support the conclusion that young people's mental health first aid knowledge and skills would benefit from improvement.

Interventions to improve mental health literacy

Surveys carried out in a number of countries, including Australia, Germany and the USA suggest that mental health literacy of a whole community can be improved (Angermeyer and Matschinger 2005; Jorm et al. 2006b; Mojtabai 2007; Goldney et al. 2009; Mojtabai 2009; Pescosolido et al. 2010). Such surveys have shown improved recognition (particularly in the case of depression) and a narrowing of the gap between the public and health professionals relating to beliefs about the helpfulness of interventions. Although it is difficult to ascribe specific causes to such changes, there is evidence that interventions to improve mental health literacy may have played a role.

Whole-of-community campaigns

There have been community campaigns in several countries that have aimed to improve aspects of mental health literacy (Dumesnil and Verger 2009). Those that have been evaluated include *beyondblue*, the Australian national government-funded depression initiative in operation since 2000. *beyondblue*'s aims include raising community understanding of depression and related disorders. *beyondblue* has used various means to achieve its aims including advertising campaigns, educating journalists, enlisting prominent people to speak about depression, sponsoring artistic and sporting events, and free information through printed materials and the internet. In its early years of operation, *beyondblue* was more active in some Australian states than others, thus allowing the lower-activity states to be used as a type of control group. Awareness of *beyondblue* was greater in members of the public in the high-activity states and there was a greater improvement in depression literacy (Jorm et al. 2005c, 2006c).

In Germany, a 2001–2002 community campaign known as the Nuremberg Alliance Against Depression (NAD), involved a public information campaign, interventions with GPs and community facilitators (for example teachers, police, clergy), and interventions with consumers and their relatives (Dietrich et al. 2009). Community surveys of mental health literacy were carried out in Nuremberg and a nearby city that had not participated in the intervention. They found that NAD increased awareness of depression, attitudes towards antidepressants became more positive and there was a decrease in the belief that depression was due to a lack of self-discipline. More importantly, there was a greater reduction in suicidal acts in Nuremberg and this change was found to persist one year after the end of the intervention (Hegerl et al. 2010). These successes led to the formation of the European Alliance Against Depression in 2004 and the extension of the approach to 17 countries.

In Norway, the Treatment and Intervention in Psychosis (TIPS) programme was designed to reduce the duration of untreated psychosis in first-episode schizophrenia (Joa et al. 2008). Run in two areas on Norway between 1997 and 2000, TIPS involved an intensive, multifaceted information campaign for the general public, schools and GPs about how to recognize psychosis, and an early detection team that could be contacted by anyone. During the intervention the median duration of untreated psychosis in the TIPS areas was five weeks, whereas in the control regions it was 16 weeks. Between 2002 and 2004 the information campaign was stopped while the early detection team continued to operate. As a result, the duration of untreated psychosis increased to a median of 15 weeks, supporting the conclusion that the information campaign was critical to the success of the intervention.

Interventions based in educational settings

Although schools have been a popular setting for mental health education interventions, relatively few have been well evaluated. A US study looked at the effects of trainee psychiatrists giving a talk to students about substance use, depression and suicide, and found an increase in willingness to seek help from a psychiatrist or counsellor (Battaglia et al. 1990). In another US study, students given a lesson about mental illness and sources of help available were more likely than a control group to show improvements in attitudes to treatment and seeking help (Esters et al. 1998). More recently, a study of a consumer-delivered educational intervention (*In Our Own Voice*) found improvements in mental health literacy at four and eight weeks' follow-up (Pinto-Foltz et al. 2011). A study in rural Pakistan looked at the effect of a four-month programme of mental health education in schools (Rahman et al. 1998). This study found improved knowledge in the school children, as well as in their parents, friends and neighbours, indicating that in a developing country a school-based programme can have a broader community impact.

Far fewer mental health literacy interventions have been carried out in higher education institutions. One recent controlled trial of a social marketing campaign with UK university students involved the use of posters and postcards to convey information about depression and its treatment (Merritt et al. 2007). Improvements were found in the recognition of depression and attitudes towards antidepressants, but no change in belief that depression can be treated effectively.

Mental health first aid training

In order to help meet the need for improved public knowledge about mental disorders, a mental health first aid training course (MHFA) was developed in Australia in 2001 (see the case study below) (Kitchener and Jorm 2008). Four randomized controlled trials have been carried out to assess the effects of the course (Jorm et al. 2004, 2010a, 2010b; Kitchener and Jorm 2004). These have all used wait-list controls and have all shown improvements in knowledge, confidence in providing help, actual helping behaviour, and stigmatizing attitudes, in particular an increased willingness to have contact with someone with a mental health problem. These changes are maintained for five to six months after course completion.

Web-based interventions

The rapid growth of the internet means that websites are now a very important source of information on mental disorders. In general, information quality is poor, although some websites, such as the US National Institute of Mental Health website (www.nimh.nih.gov), have been rated highly in several studies (Reavley and Jorm 2011b).

A number of randomized controlled trials have evaluated the effects of websites on users, including an Australian study that compared the effectiveness of a website giving information about depression and its treatment (BluePages: www.bluepages.anu.edu.au) with a website providing CBT (MoodGYM: www.moodgym.anu.edu.au) and an attention–placebo control intervention (Christensen et al. 2004). Results showed that the information website increased the participants' understanding of treatments for depression and reduced depressive symptoms although it did not improve professional help-seeking (Christensen et al. 2006). A follow-up study found these therapeutic benefits to be maintained over 12 months (Mackinnon et al. 2008). Results of such studies support the possibility that increasing mental health literacy may lead to a therapeutic benefit (Donker et al. 2009).

Web-based interventions are less likely to be accessed by people who are older, less educated and with lower incomes. This may increase health inequalities unless they are publicly funded, available in a wide range of languages and in formats that do not require literacy (Munoz 2010). Population interventions may be appropriate for most members of the community, whereas more intensive interventions will be justified for those in higher-risk groups or who are more likely to have contact with people with mental disorders. For example, MHFA has been adapted for Aboriginal and Torres Strait Islander peoples and for Vietnamese and Chinese Australians and the Australian COMPASS project had a youth focus (Wright et al. 2006).

Conclusions

Deficiencies in mental health literacy are common in many countries and limit the ability of the public to take action for prevention, early intervention, uptake of evidence-based treatment, self-help and first aid. Research conducted over the past 15 years has shown that mental disorders are generally not well recognized by the public, there are gaps between public and professional beliefs about treatment, stigma is a barrier to help-seeking and mental health first aid skills are often deficient. However, there is evidence that mental health literacy can be improved by population-level interventions and individual training programmes. Encouragingly, longitudinal studies from a number of countries suggest that improvements in mental health literacy over time have occurred.

A limitation of much of the work so far is that it has focused on beliefs rather than actions taken. Associations between beliefs and actions are modest, so there is a need to better understand the links between knowledge, attitudes and behaviour, and to show that improvements in mental health literacy can improve mental health. There is also a need to explore mental health literacy in populations that have models of mental health that may differ from those commonly seen in Western countries.

The ultimate aim of work on mental health literacy is a society in which people take appropriate action to prevent mental disorders in themselves and their families, but if they do develop a disorder, they obtain timely professional help, receive and adhere to evidence-based treatments, feel supported by those in their social network, and consequently recover more quickly.

Mini toolkit

Tips for effective practice

- Information campaigns should be intensive and multifaceted if they are to change knowledge and attitudes.
- Programmes that build on familiar models, fulfil a public need, are tailored to meet different needs, have a strong partnership with research, have procedures for quality control and have sustainable funding models are more likely to succeed.

Case study

One possible approach to improving mental health literacy is to widen the base of people with some knowledge and skills in helping people with mental health problems. Mental Health First Aid (MHFA) training is an example of such an approach. The philosophy behind MHFA is that while people with mental health problems can potentially be assisted by those in their social network, potential helpers often lack the confidence and skills to provide basic help. The MHFA course follows the model that has been successfully applied with first aid for physical disorders. It trains members of the public to give early help to people with developing mental health problems and to give assistance in mental health crisis situations. The Mental Health First Aid training course has been widely disseminated in Australia and has now reached 1 per cent of the adult population (Jorm and Kitchener 2011). The course has also been disseminated internationally and has been adapted to the culture and healthcare systems of 15 other countries (Jorm and Kitchener 2011).

Undertaking research and evaluation

- Evaluation should be theory-driven and evaluation data should be collected from the very early stages of programme development and implementation. Research should also guide the content of training, e.g. in the absence of a solid evidence base in certain areas, guidelines formulated through expert consensus were used in the development of MHFA training.

- Challenges in evaluation in this area include assessing the impact of interventions on behaviour change, particularly in the longer term, and assessing differential impacts according to participants' varying backgrounds.

Reflection points and questions

- Promising approaches to improving mental health literacy include whole-of-community campaigns, school-based interventions and mental health first-aid training. Such interventions have been shown to improve recognition of disorders and have also resulted in beliefs about treatments and causes moving closer to those of health professionals.
- Evidence that whole-of-community campaigns can increase help-seeking behaviours and reduce stigmatizing attitudes towards those with mental disorders remains weak.

Further reading and resources

- Beyondblue: www.beyondblue.org.au (accessed 23 August 2012).
- Mental Health First Aid: www.mhfa.com.au (accessed 23 August 2012).

7 Suicide prevention

Annette L Beautrais and Gregory Luke Larkin

Introduction

Suicide is a leading public health problem, and the human and economic disease burden associated with suicide is growing in both the developed and developing world (WHO 2001). The purpose of this chapter is to describe the magnitude of the problem of suicide as a global public health issue and challenge, and to outline public health approaches that may help to stem the rising tide of suicide.

Global burden

Each year an estimated one million people worldwide die by suicide, generating a global suicide rate of approximately 16 per 100,000 persons per year, and accounting for 1.5 per cent of all world deaths (WHO 2001). Suicide is the tenth leading cause of death in the world, the leading cause of violent deaths, and in some countries the third leading cause of death among 15- to 44-year-olds (WHO 2012) and, as in the UK, the second leading cause of death in 10- to 24-year-olds (Samaritans 2012). Despite an unprecedented volume of research during the past three decades exploring aetiology, risk factors and treatments for suicidal behaviour, and despite the greatest investment in suicide prevention that has ever occurred, suicide deaths are predicted to rise to 1.5 million worldwide by 2020 (WHO 2001).

In addition to suicide deaths, an estimated 9 per cent of people report having serious thoughts of suicide in their lifetime and 3 per cent report making a suicide attempt (Nock et al. 2008a, 2008b). The associated costs in terms of both years of potential life lost (YPLL) due to premature mortality and the years of productive life lost due to disability (also known as disability adjusted life years, DALYs) are profound. In addition, the healthcare and social costs associated with suicide are immense. In 2002 the US Institute of Medicine estimated the annual cost of 30,000 suicides each year to be $11.8 billion (Institute of Medicine 2002). Extrapolating from this figure, the economic costs of global suicide deaths must surely now approach $500 billion a year. The personal costs of emotional distress and suffering for the people exposed to suicidal behaviour are incalculable.

On the basis of magnitude, public health prioritization of suicide prevention is justified. Yet suicide remains a hidden public health problem, one which is undercounted, underrecognized, underfunded and non-prioritized. Even in the face of rising suicide rates, for example, suicide is not included in the 2011 announcement of the 40 priorities of the Grand Challenges of Global Mental Health, an influential initiative funded by the US National Institute of Mental Health (NIMH), supported by the Global Alliance for Chronic Diseases (GACD), headquartered in London (Collins et al. 2011).

Part of the failure to confront suicide prevention, is that ownership of the problem of suicide is now, and has historically been, very diffuse. Oft-repeated assertions that suicide prevention is 'everybody's business' convey that suicide prevention is no-one's specific responsibility. Similarly, the claim that suicide is 'a complex problem with multiple causes' implies it is a problem too complicated to solve, and impossibly difficult to address or to avert. Another barrier is the ubiquitous fatalism in the profession, even among psychiatrists, suggesting that some people will kill themselves, no matter what we do. A lack of effective suicide prevention programmes reinforces this view, often buttressed by the reluctance of government leadership to take accountability for a highly emotive issue that is seen as a political 'loser'.

Historical, cultural and social perspectives of suicide

There are a host of cultural, social and historical reasons that may explain the failure to prioritize suicide prevention as a public health issue. Suicide is prohibited in most religions, and this stance was traditionally reinforced by legal sanctions against suicide in many jurisdictions (Wasserman and Wasserman 2009). Suicide has been decriminalized only relatively recently in many countries, in England and Wales, for example, in 1961, and in Ireland in 1993, and still remains a criminal offence in some countries, such as Pakistan. The criminal connotations of suicide have pervaded and inhibited many aspects of suicide prevention, surrounding the issue with shame, stigma, underascertainment and reluctance to seek help.

In addition to historical legal influences, approaches to suicide prevention have been shaped by various theories of suicidal behaviour. The most significant of these in recent history include Durkheim's view that suicide reflects lack of societal wellbeing and social cohesion, the psychological perspective that suicide is a response to personal psychological stress, and the medical approach that holds that suicide is accounted for by mental illness, with mental disorders having genetic and environmental components. Much recent suicide research has been directed by the medical perspective, and this position has led to the current domination of suicide prevention by programmes that screen for, and treat, individuals with psychiatric illness. This focus has occurred even as suicide has been promoted as a public health issue, and has led to a focus on individual suicide risk, at the expense of primary prevention.

Prevalence

There are substantial variations in suicide rates reported to the WHO by different countries. In part this variability may be accounted for by the challenges of generating accurate, adequate and timely suicide data from countries that are highly populated, and from those in which suicide is stigmatized, criminalized, penalized or not prioritized.

Determinations of deaths as suicides, and systems for registering and reporting suicide deaths, differ among countries. In some countries a fraction of suicides are unreported, estimated, for example, in China, to be of the order of 15 per cent (Phillips et al. 2002), whereas in other countries suicides are undercounted. In Tamil Nadu, India, for example, use of trained lay interviewers to conduct 'verbal autopsy' interviews with family members generated suicide rates that were ten times higher than those reported officially to the WHO (Gajalakshmi and Peto 2007). Another source of undercounting is misclassification: Some countries may record suicides as undetermined deaths, 'open verdicts' or deaths due to accident or illness, whereas other jurisdictions may not permit these categorizations.

These various sources of underestimation have their origin in historical, social, religious, cultural, political and legal beliefs and practices about suicide. Collectively, these biases probably operate to undercount suicide substantially: Global suicide deaths may, in fact, be much higher than the near one million currently estimated. Indeed, the 1.5 million suicides projected for 2020 is also likely to be a significant underestimate.

As currently reported to the WHO, suicide rates are highest in Eastern European countries including Lithuania, Estonia, Belarus and the Russian Federation. These countries have suicide rates of the order of 45 to 75 per 100,000. By contrast, reported suicide rates are lowest in the countries of Mediterranean Europe and the predominantly Catholic countries of Latin America (Colombia, Paraguay) and Asia (for example the Philippines) and in Muslim countries (such as Pakistan). These countries have suicide rates of less than 6 per 100,000. In the developed countries of Europe, North America and Australasia suicide rates tend to lie between these two extremes, ranging from 10 to 35 per 100,000. Suicide data are not yet readily available from many countries in Africa and South America (WHO 2001, 2012).

Trends

The inadequacies and inconsistencies of national suicide reporting systems impose serious constraints on efforts to examine suicide trends, both within countries and cross-nationally. Bearing these constraints in mind, the following broad observations apply: suicide is more common in males than females in almost every country, often by a factor of 3:1 to 4:1; females make more suicide attempts than males; rates of youth suicide increased in many developed countries during the 1980s, and increased in young adults in the first decade of the twenty-first century; traditionally, older males have been most vulnerable to suicide and the current ageing of the population suggests suicide rates and numbers among the elderly will increase.

Epidemiology

In addition to underestimation, one of the challenges of suicide research has been a dearth of studies of sufficient size to examine prevalence and prediction for this low base-rate behaviour. The recent epidemiological studies of the WHO World Mental Health Surveys provide findings from large representative samples for 10 developed and 11 developing countries for a total study population of 108,000 (Kessler and Ustun 2008; Nock et al. 2008a; Borges et al. 2010). Cross-national comparisons generated 12-month prevalence estimates of suicidal behaviour that were very similar for both developed and developing countries. Specifically, rates of suicide ideation, plans and attempts were 2.0 per cent, 0.6 per cent and 0.3 per cent respectively for developed countries and 2.1 per cent, 0.7 per cent and 0.4 per cent for developing countries (Borges et al. 2010).

These studies also showed that the risk factors for suicidal behaviour, as assessed in this survey, were similar in both developed and developing countries, and included: female gender, younger age, lower education and income, unmarried status, unemployment, parental psychopathology, childhood adversity, presence of a wide range of (DSM-IV) mental disorders in the previous year, and psychiatric comorbidity (Borges et al. 2010). These risk factors were associated with suicide attempts because they predicted suicide ideation. Combining these risk factors, it was possible to generate a risk index that accurately predicted 12-month suicide attempts (area under the curve (AUC)=0.74–0.80).

More specifically, these WHO-sponsored studies found that, controlling for psychiatric comorbidity, anxiety disorders and impulse–control disorders predicted which people among those with suicide ideation would make suicide attempts. Overall, mental disorders were equally predictive of suicide attempt in both developed and developing countries. However, the strongest predictors of suicide attempt in developed countries were mood disorders, whereas the strongest predictors in developing countries were substance-use disorders, impulse–control disorders and PTSD (Nock et al. 2008a).

Findings from global studies highlight the fact that suicidal behaviour is a complex phenomenon and, usually, no single cause is sufficient to explain a suicidal act. During the past three decades an extensive body of knowledge has accumulated about the biological, cultural, social, psychological and contextual factors that can influence risk of suicidal behaviour.

There is a remarkable consistency, across cultures and countries, in the micro-level risk factors for suicide identified in these studies (Institute of Medicine 2002). Risk of suicide can be influenced by individual vulnerability or resiliency related to age, gender, ethnicity, religious values, genetic and biological factors, personality traits, sexual orientation and immigrant status. People from socially, economically and educationally disadvantaged backgrounds are at increased risk of suicidal behaviour. Childhood adversity and trauma, and various life stresses as an adult influence risks of suicidal behaviour.

Suicide risk is elevated for all mental disorders except for learning disability and dementia (Harris and Barraclough 1997). In particular, mood disorders, substance use disorders, anxiety disorders, impulse–control disorders, and schizophrenia and other psychotic disorders, all increase risk of suicide. Hopelessness elevates suicide risk independently of mental disorder. Diminished social interaction and lack of social connectedness increase suicide risk, particularly among adults and older adults.

At the macro (population) level, social cohesion and integration protect against suicide. The ready availability of means of suicide (for example, firearms or pesticides) or access to suicide 'hotspots' (sites with reputations for suicide) increases the risk that suicidal ideation will be converted to a suicide death. Media reporting practices that glamorize suicide or gratuitously cover celebrity suicides, unusual methods of suicide or suicide clusters risk promoting contagion and suicides among vulnerable individuals.

All of these micro- and macro-level risk factors tend to act cumulatively to increase suicide risk. The fact that there are multiple pathways to suicidal behaviour, and the absence of a single, readily identifiable high-risk group accounting for the majority of suicides, imply that many different types of programmes and activities are needed to prevent suicide. Each programme and action may contribute to reducing suicide. Figure 7.1 summarizes the extensive body of research about the individual, genetic, psychiatric, social, cultural and contextual ecology of suicidal behaviour, and links these risk factors with opportunities to intervene at the micro-, meso- and macro-levels to reduce the likelihood of suicidal behaviour.

A public health approach to suicide prevention

Suicide is commonly defined as a public health problem, and a public health approach underpins most national suicide prevention strategies (Jenkins 2002; Knox et al. 2004; Beautrais 2005). The public health approach to a health issue encompasses surveillance, the formulation

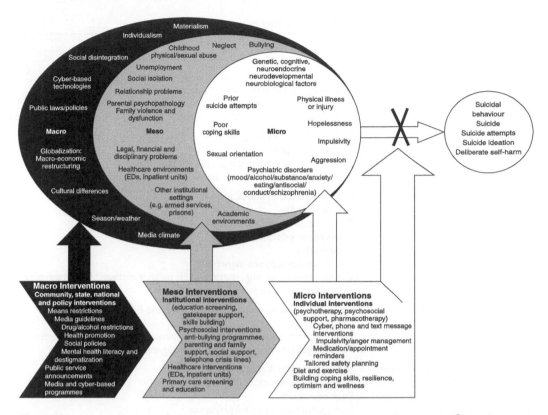

Figure 7.1 An ecological model of suicide risk and prevention. ED, emergency department. © A.L. Beautrais and G.L. Larkin.

of public policies to address identified local and national health problems and priorities, and the promotion of cost-effective healthcare policies for at-risk populations. Table 7.1 summarizes the broad range of sites and settings available for suicide prevention.

Adopting a public health framework, national suicide prevention plans typically include a wide range of strategies in efforts to:

- control access to means of suicide;
- enhance training, recognition, assessment, treatment and management of depression by medical practitioners, particularly in primary care;
- increase public awareness of depression by programmes that promote mental health literacy and help-seeking, and destigmatize mental illness;
- improve assessment, treatment and follow-up care of people who make suicide attempts and present to emergency departments;
- enhance access to mental health services and improve the care of people with serious mental illness;
- provide targeted prevention programmes for identified high-risk populations;
- encourage responsible media reporting and portrayal of suicide;
- improve control of alcohol and other substances;

Table 7.1 Suicide prevention settings and strategies

Settings	Strategies
Individuals	Pharmacotherapy, pharmacogenomic therapy Psychological/behavioural treatments Psychosocial interventions Combinations of pharmacotherapeutic/psychological/psychosocial therapies
Families	Early intervention programmes Parenting support Support/mentorship programmes for at-risk youth Family-based therapy (e.g. multisystemic therapy, MST)
Schools and colleges	Curriculum-based education Skills building Peer education and support Gatekeeper education Case finding At-risk group support/mentoring Cyber-based screening, therapy, skills building and wellbeing promotion Combinations of strategies listed above
Healthcare systems	Emergency departments (ED) screening and ED-initiated treatment programmes General practitioner education, screening, treatment and management Hospital-based inpatient/outpatient programmes
Other institutional systems Child welfare Courts/justice Armed Forces	Screening and risk monitoring Gatekeeper education Peer education Institutional support and protocols Means restriction Skills building Treatment programmes
Communities	Community gatekeeper programmes Telephone crisis lines Active membership of religious, spiritual or some other social group Safe storage programmes for potentially lethal agents Cyber-based screening, education, treatment Media suicide reporting resources Promotion of family and community connectedness Postvention support services for those bereaved by suicide
National/state	Means restriction Mental health literacy and public education/destigmatization Promotion of mental and physical wellbeing Alcohol legislation Social welfare policies Full employment policies Adequate medical and social care

- provide crisis centres and counselling, including telephone 'hotlines';
- encourage school-based competency-promoting and skill-enhancing programmes for young people;
- provide efforts to interrupt suicide clusters, minimize contagion and support communities in which a cluster occurs;
- provide effective support for families and others bereaved by suicide;
- encourage research, evidence-based approaches to programme development, evaluation of components of the national strategy, and the production of timely and accurate statistics on suicide and attempted suicide;
- promote healthy lifestyle and population wellness programmes.

However, while national suicide prevention strategies typically propose most, if not all, of these interventions, few evaluations of their effectiveness have been conducted. Physician education in depression recognition and treatment, and restricting access to lethal methods have been shown to reduce suicide rates. All other interventions require more evaluation to demonstrate efficacy (Mann et al. 2005).

Models of public health action

A number of public health disease and injury prevention models might be applied to suicide prevention, including, for example, the primary, secondary and tertiary model of disease prevention, Gordon's three-tiered classification system of universal, selective and indicated prevention (Gordon 1987), the Haddon Matrix model of injury prevention (Haddon 1970, 1980) and Frieden's four-level model for public health action (Frieden 2010).

The Haddon Matrix is a conceptual model that illustrates how the principles of public health might be applied to understand the aetiology of suicidal behaviour and to identify potential preventive strategies (Haddon 1970, 1980). This model is based on the host (or individual person at risk), the agent or means of injury and the physical and social environment in which the injury occurs. Haddon's Matrix also includes phases at which interventions would potentially have effect (pre-event, event and post-event). Table 7.2 provides an example of the

Table 7.2 Application of Haddon's Matrix to preventing suicide by jumping from high places

	Pre-event	Event	Post-event
Host	Genetic vulnerability to suicide; mental health, prior attempts	Acute stress, intoxication, impulsivity, intent	Emergency medical services (EMS), police, emergency department (ED), access, resuscitation, medical treatment, psychiatric treatment
Agent	Bridge barriers; access; iconic status	Height of fall; impact; trauma	Barriers; other bridges nearby; engineering solutions
Environment (physical, sociocultural, legal)	Social capital; media reports; prior jumpers; acceptability	Trauma centre; emergency distress call centre; police; EMS; witnesses	Strengthen building, engineering codes; enforce media reporting guidelines; postvention support

application of Haddon's Matrix to suicide prevention, specifically, to preventing suicide by jumping from high places. A further example of the application of Haddon's Matrix to suicidal behaviour is provided by Eddleston and colleagues (2006), who used this model to identify strategies to reduce suicides by organophosphate self-poisoning.

Applied to suicide prevention, this public health perspective provides a useful framework for developing an agenda to better identify aetiological factors and at-risk populations and develop and implement new prevention programmes. For example, applied to surveillance, further research is required to: develop a consistent terminology for suicidal behaviours; enhance coding accuracy in healthcare services, morbidity and mortality records; improve the timeliness of morbidity and mortality data; identify underutilized sites and databases (such as emergency departments, child welfare populations) and extend collection of morbidity and mortality data to include more comprehensive and useful information than the ubiquitous age by gender by method comparisons. Figure 7.2 summarizes this perspective by outlining ten stakeholder groups whose contributions are vital links in the chain of suicide prevention.

Applied to epidemiological analysis, research is required to: develop suicide attempt registers for research and for monitoring at-risk populations; conduct observational studies and extend analyses beyond simple bivariate comparisons to include testing of theoretical models (such as gene-by-environment interactions) that more accurately reflect the complex multifactorial nature of suicidal behaviour; exploit new electronic medical and institutional (such as school, college) records systems to conduct longitudinal studies of outcome after suicide attempts, and of the developmental trajectories of suicidal behaviour; make use of modern computing technology and electronic records systems to conduct large multisite epidemiological surveys, utilizing novel methodological approaches to examine suicide problems (for example explore clustering of suicide attempts using geospatial mapping techniques, or use computer-based platforms to elicit anonymous information about suicidal behaviours in order to

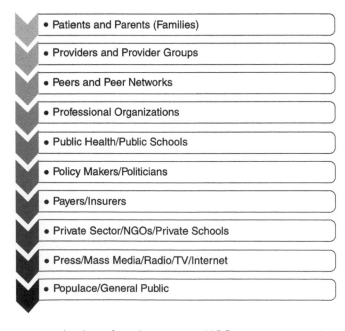

- Patients and Parents (Families)
- Providers and Provider Groups
- Peers and Peer Networks
- Professional Organizations
- Public Health/Public Schools
- Policy Makers/Politicians
- Payers/Insurers
- Private Sector/NGOs/Private Schools
- Press/Mass Media/Radio/TV/Internet
- Populace/General Public

Figure 7.2 Stakeholders in the chain of suicide prevention. NGO, non-governmental organization.

achieve more accurate information) (Tourangeau and Smith 1996; Perlis et al. 2004; Claassen and Larkin 2005).

Applied to interventions, the public health perspective includes a research agenda to develop and evaluate prevention programmes. The general principles of effective programme development and implementation are now the focus of an area that has become known as prevention science (Kellam and Langevin 2003). The key principles of programme development within the prevention science framework include: using theory and research evidence to develop promising policies and interventions; using pilot, model and demonstration programmes to determine the acceptability of a proposed programme to the targeted population, the feasibility of implementing the programme, and the safety and effectiveness of the programme; throughout the process of programme development undertaking evaluations to examine the formation of the programme, the processes by which the programme is delivered and the efficacy, effectiveness and cost-effectiveness of the programme; identifying meaningful outcome measures, and refining and identifying the critical elements of effective programmes. These critical research and evaluation elements of the prevention science approach appear most suitable for developing suicide prevention programmes.

A public health approach includes the use of true, natural and quasi-experimental approaches to examine prevention and intervention programmes. For example, the removal of safety barriers at a bridge and their subsequent reinstallation provided a natural and powerful a–b–a reversal design by which the impact of changes in access to the bridge on suicides from the bridge could be examined (Beautrais et al. 2009). Similarly, the introduction of more restrictive firearms legislation provided a naturalistic before and after study of the impact of these changes on suicides (Beautrais et al. 2006). The detoxification of domestic gas in the UK markedly reduced both suicides by that method and overall suicide rates (Kreitman 1976). Suicide rates by overdose of antidepressants fell when tricyclic antidepressants were substantially replaced by the clinically safer selective serotonin reuptake inhibitor (SSRIs) that are less toxic in overdose (Phillips et al. 1997). Quasi-experimental designs are appropriate when true experiments cannot be conducted.

Public health approaches also strongly emphasize community and legislative interventions to achieve environmental changes. Applied to suicide prevention, this perspective includes: reducing access to the means of suicide; encouraging the media to report suicide in a muted manner to minimize the risk of glamorizing suicide or of promoting specific methods of suicide; using media and social marketing techniques to destigmatize suicide and the mental illnesses with which it is associated, and decriminalizing suicide in those countries where it remains a crime. Little is known about the impact of public health messages focused on suicide but caution is warranted given the body of evidence about the deleterious impact of incautious media reporting of suicide (Chambers et al. 2005). However, mass media campaigns and community interventions to promote healthy lifestyles have made highly successful contributions to address complex public health problems such as cardiovascular disease (Sanddal et al. 2003; Knox et al. 2004). The extent to which carefully crafted and monitored similar interventions could promote individual wellness and support communities to improve population mental health, and thereby address the complex public health problem of suicide, is a matter for much research.

Development of relevant policy and dissemination of new findings are key components of a public health approach. Translational research is the means by which new findings are communicated and implemented. A research agenda in this area includes examining barriers and access to healthcare and preventive services, assessing service quality and costs of new services, and determining the optimal ways in which to disseminate and implement new programmes (Larkin et al. 2007; Insel 2009).

For suicide prevention a critical component of translational research is the creation of new types of organizational and administrative structures that permit the development and implementation of suicide prevention programmes: whereas variants of the funder/provider model (in which funders let contracts to various providers) work well for the purchase of well-defined services from expert providers, this model is less appropriate where there is a need to develop and evaluate new programmes or services. Since the field of suicide prevention lacks both evidence-based intervention programmes, and expert providers, the field will rely increasingly upon new structures that will fund and support the development and evaluation of effective prevention programmes (MacQueen and Cates 2005).

As new suicide prevention programmes are developed, a critical task for public health policy and translational research is to develop standards for identifying effective prevention programmes and policies that are ready for dissemination, in order to inform the field and to populate it with prevention programmes and policies of proven efficacy, effectiveness or readiness for adoption (Flay et al. 2005). This knowledge translation activity is particularly salient for suicide prevention since it is an emotive area in which there is a risk of iatrogenic effects from poorly evaluated interventions delivered by well-intended providers who may lack experience and expertise in the suicide field. More generally, this issue highlights the need for the establishment of an educated, expert and experienced suicide prevention research and practitioner workforce with the capacity to develop, implement and evaluate new programmes. Education is an essential component of a public health approach to address the current challenge facing suicide prevention, i.e. of bridging the gap between basic knowledge about the causes of suicide and the development of effective population-based programmes and policies.

Since suicidal behaviours are often the endpoint of a complex series of interrelated factors, a wide range of social, educational and health policies may potentially contribute to suicide prevention. However, it is important to place the role of such policies in context: the policy focus in many areas will be on addressing a wide range of public health and social issues, and suicide prevention will often be a secondary goal. For example, the reduction of violence is the primary objective of family violence policy and any reduction of suicidal behaviours is secondary to that objective. Second, it is likely that because of the complex causation of suicidal behaviours the contribution of any single specific policy to reducing rates of suicidal behaviour in the population will be small. Nonetheless, although the contributions of single policies to suicide prevention may be modest, the collective contributions of a portfolio of policies addressing a broad range of health, social and contextual factors related to suicidal behaviours may be substantial.

Conclusions

This chapter outlined the epidemiology of suicide, and public health approaches that could be implemented to address this global problem. In response to UN and WHO counsel that individual countries should develop national suicide prevention policies, linked where possible to other public health programmes, an increasing number of countries have developed national suicide prevention plans. Generally these plans have adopted a public health framework. Commonly, implementation of these plans has seen investments weighted in favour of individual-level psychiatric treatments, and community investment in gatekeeper training and school-based programmes, for which, despite their intuitive appeal, there is no evidence of effectiveness. To date, suicide prevention efforts have been parochial, and primary prevention has been relatively neglected. Suicide rates have not decreased and are projected to rise. This forecast suggests that it is time to adopt a wider lens for suicide prevention, and to implement population-level strategies that address societal influences and inequalities in the contexts in which suicide occurs. A public health model provides a framework for action for the armamentarium of approaches needed to address suicide prevention. As the US Institute of

Medicine opined ten years ago: 'If ever a condition begged for an integrated understanding that takes into account biological, clinical, subjective, and social factors, this is it' (Institute of Medicine 2002: i).

Mini toolkit

Tips for effective practice

In this complex area, the following papers include evidence-based public health models and developing effective models and practice.

- Frieden, T.R. (2010) A framework for public health action: the health impact pyramid, *American Journal of Public Health*, 100: 590–595.
- Jenkins, R. (2002) Addressing suicide as a public-health problem, *Lancet*, 359: 813–814.
- Knox, K.L., Conwell, Y. and Caine, E.D. (2004) If suicide is a public health problem, what are we doing to prevent it?, *American Journal of Public Health*, 94: 37–45.
- Knox, K.L., Pflanz, S., Talcott, G.W., Campise, R.L., Lavigne, J.E., Bajorska, A., Tu, X. and Caine, E.D. (2010) The US Air Force suicide prevention program: implications for public health policy, *American Journal of Public Health*, 100: 2457–2463.
- MacQueen, K. and Cates, W. (2005) The multiple layers of prevention science research, *American Journal of Preventive Medicine*, 28: 491–495.

Case study

An example of a national public health programme to reduce suicide is 'Talk To Me', the national action plan to reduce suicide and self-harm in Wales. The programme is running from 2008 to 2013 and details on the programme can be found at www.wales.gov.uk/consultations/healthsocialcare/talktome.

Undertaking research and evaluation

To learn more about conducting research and evaluation in suicide prevention see the following.

- Flay, B.R., Biglan, A., Boruch, R.F., Castro, F.G., Gottfredson, D., Kellam, S., Moscicki, E.K., Schinke, S., Valentine, J.C. and Ji, P. (2005) Standards of evidence: Criteria for efficacy, effectiveness and dissemination, *Prevention Science*, 6: 151–175.
- Kellam, S.G. and Langevin, D.J. (2003) A framework for understanding 'evidence' in prevention research and programs, *Prevention Science*, 4: 137–153.

Reflection points and questions

- Are there examples of the successful adoption of a public health approach to address a medical or social problem of complex multidisciplinary aetiology that provide appropriate models for suicide prevention?
- To what extent is it possible to achieve control of a public health problem when the aetiology and epidemiology are not clear (for example taking the pump handle off to control consumption of water thought to be the aetiological vehicle of cholera)?
- How might Frieden's framework for public health action be applied to suicide prevention?

Further reading and resources

Further information can be found in the following publications and resources.

- Hawton, K. and van Heeringen, K. (2009) Suicide, *Lancet*, 373: 1372–1381.
- Nock, M.K., Borges, G., Bromet, E.J., Cha, C.B., Kessler, R.C. and Lee, S. (2008) Suicide and suicidal behavior, *Epidemiologic Reviews*, 30: 133–154.
- WHO suicide data available at: www.who.int/mental_health/prevention/suicide/country_reports/en/index.html (accessed 24 August 2012).

8 Preventing depression

Margaret Maxwell

Introduction

This chapter focuses on preventing common mental health problems that mainly comprise of depression and anxiety-related disorders. Depression and anxiety can be classified as mild, moderate or severe depending on the severity of symptoms and their impact on an individual's daily life. These common mental health problems cause significant distress and interfere with daily function but do not include psychotic symptoms. There are more specific types of depression and anxiety such as bipolar disorder, postnatal depression, seasonal affective disorder (SAD), phobias and obsessive–compulsive disorder. These specific disorders are not addressed in this chapter, although some may at times have been included in some authors' definitions of common mental disorders.

Overview of public health burden

For over a decade we have become familiar with the scale and impact of common mental health problems worldwide. Data from WHO predictions on the global burden of illness have placed depression as becoming the second leading cause of disability worldwide (Murray and Lopez 1997). It is estimated that depression affects between 5 and 10 per cent of the world's population at any given time. In the UK, a national survey of psychiatric morbidity found that 16.2 per cent of adults met the diagnostic criteria for at least one common mental disorder in the week prior to interview. More than half of those with a common mental disorder presented with mixed anxiety and depressive disorder (9 per cent) (NHS Information Centre for Health and Social Care 2009). Annually, 6–8 per cent of adults have an episode of depression, and more than 15 per cent (estimates include up to 25 per cent) of the population will experience an episode during their lifetime (Wang et al. 2003).

Estimates of common mental health problems can vary because of differences in definition as to what constitutes a diagnosis of depression (the prevalence of major depression disorder) and what might constitute subthreshold depression and low mood. The latter is more common but together they represent the range of problems that are mostly managed within primary care. It is estimated common mental health problems are the third most common reason for a consultation in primary care, and that one-third of consultations have a mental health component (Gilbody et al. 2003).

Economic burden

The economic burden of depression has also received much attention in recent years, and although different estimates are provided depending on the countries involved and the methods of calculation, it is generally accepted that the costs to society are huge, running to tens of billions of dollars in the USA alone, and largely attributable to the loss of work productivity (Greenberg et al. 2003b). In the UK, the total loss of output due to depression and chronic anxiety is estimated at some £12 billion a year or 1 per cent of total national income (Centre for Economic Performance's Mental Health Policy Group 2006). Worldwide some 40 per cent of all disability (physical and mental) is due to mental illness, and as a reflection of this, 40 per cent of people on Incapacity Benefits in the UK are in receipt of these because of mental illness (Oxford Economics 2007).

Taking together, the prevalence, burden and economic costs of depression indicate that preventing depression is a major public health issue. Understanding the risk factors for depression should then facilitate the introduction of appropriate strategies and interventions that lead to prevention of illness.

Risk factors

Depression is likely to result from a complex interaction of biological, psychological and social factors (NICE 2009a). A review of current evidence on biological markers for depression (focusing on neurotrophic factors, serotonergic markers, biochemical markers, immunological markers, neuroimaging, neurophysiological findings and neuropsychological markers) found there were no biological markers currently available for major depression (Moessner et al. 2007). The presence of chronic physical health problems such as diabetes, chronic obstructive pulmonary disease and cardiovascular disease also make depression more likely but the direction of any causal relationship between chronic illness and depression remains generally unexplained.

Psychological theories relate to three main schools of thought: psychodynamic (where unconscious conflicts from loss or grief impact on the self); cognitive (negative thinking); and behavioural (learned helplessness). These can be expressed as predisposing personality traits, and through variations in responses to stress mechanisms (diathesis-stress model). However, it is the interplay between psychological and environmental/social issues (such as poverty/social deprivation, unemployment, living alone) that show most promise in understanding the risk factors for depression and for intervening at both individual and societal/community levels.

The ONS Survey of Psychiatric Morbidity conducted in the UK allows further understanding of the social risk factors associated with the prevalence of common mental disorders (NHS Information Centre for Health and Social Care 2009). This study has reported that those identified with symptoms indicating common mental disorder (in the past week) are more likely (than those without) to be:

- women (19.7 per cent for women versus 12.5 per cent for men);
- aged between 45 and 54 for women, and aged between 25 and 54 for men;

- not married or widowed;
- living in households with the lowest levels of income.

In terms of ethnicity, the ONS survey found little variation between White, Black and South Asian men in the rates of any common mental disorder. However, among women, rates of all common mental disorders (except phobias) were higher in the South Asian group. Although the sample size of Asian women in the ONS survey was relatively small ($n=90$), they represent a potential high-risk group (in Western/European cultures) as a focus for intervention.

From further studies other known associations with potential risk factors include work-related stress, poor housing, negative life events, a family history of depression, presence of other mental health problems (such as schizophrenia or dementia), social isolation and lack of confiding relationships, and problems with alcohol (Bruce and Hoff 1994; Salokangas and Poutanen 1998; Weich and Lewis 1998; Stansfeld et al. 1999; Angst et al. 2003).

With such an array of potential causes and risk factors (and for many individuals there will likely be multiple risk factors at play) it is difficult to know which risk factors to prioritize within prevention activities. A multifactor risk algorithm to predict major depression has recently been published, with a similar algorithm for anxiety to follow, and these may influence future prevention efforts in primary care (King et al. 2008). This risk algorithm included the following risk factors: age, sex, educational level achieved, results of lifetime screen for depression, family history of psychological difficulties, physical health and mental health subscale scores on the Short Form-12, unsupported difficulties in paid or unpaid work, and experiences of discrimination.

Prognosis

Although 50 per cent of depressive episodes that people experience improve without any medical intervention, it is also understood that depression is likely to recur in the majority of cases (Timonen and Liukkonen 2008). Approximately 80 per cent of people who have received psychiatric care for an episode of depression will have at least one more episode in their lifetime (with a median of four episodes). In primary care only about one-third of patients will remain well at 11 years following an episode of depression, and about 20 per cent will experience chronic recurrent depression (Katon and Schulberg 1992; Kessler et al. 2003). Risk factors for increased risk of depression recurrence include:

- three or more previous episodes of major depression;
- high prior frequency of recurrence;
- an episode in the previous 12 months;
- residual symptoms during continuation treatment;
- severe episodes, for example 'suicidality', psychotic features;
- long previous episodes;
- relapse after drug discontinuation (NHS Clinical Knowledge Summaries (2011).

Early recognition and intervention

In the absence of the availability of interventions for the prevention of onset of common mental health problems, the emphasis has been placed on earlier recognition and intervention. Early recognition includes screening for depression, either in the general population (as has previously been advocated within the USA) or in known high-risk groups such as those with long-term physical illness (as advocated in the UK) (Boersma and Linton 2005; NICE 2009a, 2009b). In 2002, the US Preventive Services Task Force (USPSTF) recommended screening adults for depression in clinical practices that have systems in place to assure accurate diagnosis, effective treatment, and follow-up (Pignone et al. 2002). This has recently been updated to conclude that screening programmes without staff-assisted depression care supports are unlikely to improve depression outcomes, although depression treatment can be effective in adults of all ages (O'Connor et al. 2009). However, other reviews have concluded that screening is not effective for improving outcomes of depression (Coyne et al. 2003; Gilbody et al. 2005; Thombs et al. 2011). Evidence of the longer-term impact of routine screening programmes is limited. The UK NHS introduced annual screening for depression in patients with diabetes and coronary heart disease as part of the General Practice Quality and Outcomes Framework (QOF) contract (Department of Health 2011b). An audit of this depression screening in general practice in the UK found that it resulted in very few new diagnoses of depression (Subramanian and Hopayian 2008) and there is a general lack of support for the use of screening tools in primary care (Dowrick et al. 2009).

When screening is promoted, some studies recommend the routine use of a screening questionnaire using two short questions (also referred to as the Whooley questions), to detect depression in those known to be at higher risk (Whooley et al. 1997; Hickie et al. 2002). These populations include people who have diabetes, coronary heart disease, and women during and after pregnancy. If people score positively for these two questions (see mini toolkit below) they may have depression and further evaluation using the Patient Health Questionnaire (PHQ-9), the Hospital Anxiety and Depression Scale (HADS) or the Beck Depression Inventory (BDI-II) is recommended (Beck et al. 1961; Zigmond and Snaith 1983; Beck et al. 1996; Spitzer et al. 1999; NICE 2009a, 2009b).

However, there is yet to be a universally agreed set of criteria for the diagnosis of depression and one that can adequately or unequivocally distinguish between severe, moderate and mild depression. A recent study of screening tools used in primary care demonstrated that the PHQ-9 and the HADS differed considerably in how they categorized severity of depression (Cameron et al. 2008). General practitioners are most often managing subthreshold disorders that do not meet formal diagnostic criteria but which nonetheless represent significant levels of impairment. Such problems can be relatively short lived and transient, or longer term (such as dysthymia). Many doctors also recognize that it is the life circumstances of patients that contribute to their distress. What is required is a more holistic assessment of need that does not focus solely on diagnosis but which also takes account of functional status/disability, duration and chronicity of symptoms, and any underlying social or physical problems.

Treatment of mild-to-moderate depression/common mental health problems

The treatment and management of common mental health problems places a very high burden on primary care. Treatment options are currently largely confined to medication (which are not recommended as a first-line response for mild to moderate depression and anxiety) and psychotherapeutic treatments (where demand and high waiting lists prohibit such responses for large numbers of patients).

The response in many Western healthcare systems has been to introduce lower intensity non-pharmacological treatments and to increase the intensity of intervention as required. This is known as 'stepped care' (see Figure 8.1). In line with stepped care, the collaborative care model has also been developed to improve the management of depression. Collaborative care models normally apply to those with more severe depression who require more intensive management within primary care. Evidence from organizational models of care has demonstrated that stepped-care and collaborative-care models are effective in delivering integrated care, in ways

Step 4	Specialist services including: specialist perinatal mental health team; eating disorders; psychoanalytical psychotherapy; inpatient services	Meeting the needs of people, and their carers and significant others, with long-standing and/or complex mental health problems requiring acute, ongoing or intensive support, care and treatment
Step 3	Secondary care services including community mental health teams; community substance misuse services; community rehabilitation team	Meeting the needs of people with long-standing and/or complex mental health problems requiring acute, ongoing or intensive support, care and treatment, and for prevention of relapse. Provision within the community
Step 2	Primary healthcare: including family practice and primary care mental health services	Meeting the needs of people experiencing mental distress, emotional problems and poor mental health caused by distressing life events and transitions; trauma and physical health problems
Step 1	Communities and local neighbourhoods	Preventing the onset of mental health problems or minimizing the impact of mental health problems in high-risk groups. Raising communities' awareness of psychosocial aspects of mental health and their impact
Step 0	Education and public awareness	Raising the level of mental health literacy in the general population; education and awareness; promotion of strategies to prevent mental ill health

Figure 8.1 Example of a stepped-care model that includes community level supports.

which best meets the needs of individuals (Katon et al. 1995, 1996, 1999; Von Korff and Goldberg 2001; Bower et al. 2006).

In general, care is 'stepped' in intensity, beginning with limited professional input through to specialist care. Some models include steps at the level of the community and prior to any medical involvement. Many stepped-care approaches or service developments aim to increase provision at the lower levels as this can be a cost-effective way to improve access to treatment, and one that does not appear to overload specialist mental health services.

In the UK NICE guidelines also concur with this stepped-care treatment model: they recommend watchful waiting, with further assessment normally within two weeks. The first step in terms of interventions would be low-intensity psychosocial and self-help interventions, chosen according to patient preference (for example: exercise, brief CBT, computerized or internet-based CBT), with the recommendation that guided self-help is best (NICE 2006, 2009a).

The 'Improving Access to Psychological Therapies' initiative in England is an example of a national programme to implement stepped-care provision for depression that includes provision of a variety of guided self-help interventions and brief CBT delivery (Department of Health 2008; Gyani et al. 2011).

Guided self-help

Guided self-help involves the role of a 'therapist' in delivering the self-help module to the patient (or client) and who will also monitor the progress of the patient/client. There are many variations of this model, depending on the type and level of qualifications of the 'therapists' delivering the self-help materials: which may include the use of non-qualified self-help workers through to clinical psychologists and psychiatrists supporting the delivery of CBT-based self-help approaches.

The evidence base for brief CBT interventions and CBT self-help interventions is strong (Churchill et al. 2001; Department of Health 2001a; Cuijpers et al. 2009; NICE 2009a). However, trials in primary care report higher attrition rates and especially among those from lower socioeconomic backgrounds (Tognoni et al. 1991; Fairhurst and Dowrick 1996; Wilson et al. 2000). Psychotherapies (including CBT-based treatments) aim to change individual behaviour and thinking patterns and do not attend to the social origins which cause or exacerbate many mental health problems. The ability to engage with, and therefore the effectiveness, of CBT-based interventions in people living in challenging social circumstances may be limited.

The future direction for the management of most chronic illnesses is based on patient involvement and active participation in their care, particularly through the encouragement of self-care/self-management mechanisms. The 'disease and treatment model' alone is unlikely to meet the complex needs associated with, and the underlying causes of depression. A more holistic view encompassing mental, physical and social needs is required.

Use of antidepressants

Evidence reviewed within NICE does not generally support the use of pharmacological treatments for people suffering from mild to moderate depression (NICE 2009a). Antidepressants are *not* recommended for the initial treatment of mild depression, because the risk–benefit ratio is poor. There is also emerging evidence surrounding the substantial placebo effects of antidepressant medication and that neither new nor older antidepressants are consistently distinguishable from placebo, and the superiority sometimes observed may be attributable to non-specific effects or other methodological artefacts (Kirsch and Sapirstein 1998; Walsh et al. 2002; Lima and Moncrief 2003; Gartlehner et al. 2008; Kirsch et al. 2008; Cipriani et al. 2009; Fournier et al. 2010). There is also general reluctance among patient populations in using antidepressants, with most patients preferring to engage in 'talking therapies' (Kessing et al. 2005; Maxwell 2005; Turner et al. 2008).

Medication management support, such as in the collaborative-care model, is more appropriate for those with moderate to severe depression in receipt of antidepressant medication. This helps to encourage adherence to the prescribed dosage and use of antidepressants as well as closer monitoring of outcomes so that appropriate changes to medications can be made if required. As debates surrounding the efficacy of antidepressants continue, efforts to include alternative management strategies should be increased.

Promotion and prevention activities: self-help and lifestyle interventions

It is now widely understood that social, economic and environmental factors have a significant influence on the mental health and wellbeing of people. Social prescribing (or social referral) is a means for linking patients in primary care with non-medical sources of support within the community that can help alleviate mental health problems or help to deal with some of the potential causes of mental distress (Department of Health 2001b). These might include opportunities for arts and creativity, physical activity, learning and volunteering, mutual aid, befriending and self-help, as well as support with social security benefits, housing, debt, employment, legal advice or parenting skills.

Social prescribing is perceived to have a number of positive outcomes for people experiencing mild to moderate mental health problems. These outcomes include:

- enhanced self-esteem and reduced low mood;
- opportunities for social contact;
- increased self-efficacy;
- transferable skills;
- greater confidence.

Although the evidence base for social prescribing is emerging, it is potentially helpful as an adjunct, or alternative, to medication or psychological interventions or as a method of supporting the psychosocial needs of vulnerable populations. However, there are also problems surrounding the up-take of these alternative interventions by healthcare professionals. Cultural differences between medical and community development models may be a potential barrier to promoting social prescribing. At the same time, social prescribing fits well as a commitment to increasing patient choice and to addressing the social and economic determinants of health. Psychosocial needs and social inclusion can be better met by access to community and voluntary resources, and facilitated through models of service delivery between primary care and the community.

Mini toolkit

Tips for effective practice

Key to mental health promotion and prevention of common mental health problems is awareness raising of mental health and its determinants among healthcare professionals. This will facilitate the use of social and psychosocial interventions to promote mental well-being and to manage problems at the mild to moderate stage when lower intensity and non-medical interventions can help.

Screening for at-risk populations could be addressed through more holistic assessment of patients needs that considers their symptoms (and severity) alongside their functional status, wider social circumstances, lifestyle and life events.

Having access to a wider range of psychological and social/community-based supports can help to manage both the symptoms (through brief CBT interventions for example) and also address wider issues that may cause or exacerbate common mental health problems. Guided self-help interventions for mild to moderate problems can also improve self-efficacy, help develop coping strategies and build confidence and self-esteem.

Case studies

The NHS in England have developed 'Increasing Access to Psychological Therapies', to ensure people with anxiety and depression have free, timely access to evidence-based psychological 'talking' therapies in primary care. Evidence indicates savings through reduced demand for stepped up care and drugs, lowered public costs and greater recovery and employability. Over 3,000 practitioners have been trained and treated over 600,000 people (www.iapt.nhs.uk).

'Steps for Stress' is an innovative primary care mental health service based on stepped-care principles but with emphasis on promotion and prevention and accessibility for disadvantaged groups. Their flexible range of activities includes individual therapy, advice clinics, phone line, stress awareness classes, support groups and book prescriptions. Practitioners undertake awareness work in local schools and communities using diverse media including films and comedy to make their messages accessible (www.glasgowsteps.com).

Undertaking research and evaluation

Contributing to the evidence base surrounding social- and community-based interventions can be problematic. The gold-standard randomised controlled trial (RCT) design (promoted within psychiatry and psychology) is not always achievable. People often expect a degree of anonymity when approaching voluntary services and are more reluctant to feel they are being monitored (for outcomes). The fact that they have already sought help from these services makes randomization to receive no intervention or a dummy intervention ethically problematic for those providing help. Even if an RCT design was possible, there is the added difficulty in demonstrating a positive (or negative) effect in mild or subthreshold populations without recruiting very large numbers of participants – hence most trials of interventions are with individuals with major depressive disorder.

The problem of bias in populations that are selected to participate in trials also needs to be addressed (for example, they often exclude people with additional complexity such as problems with alcohol and drug misuse, communication problems, people who may have difficulty with the self-motivation required for CBT interventions). Solutions are required that combat poor up-take and attrition among economically disadvantaged populations, although this may already be alleviated through researching interventions that may be more acceptable to such groups.

Reflection points and questions

- Are current diagnostic criteria helpful?
- Is screening for depression worthwhile?
- What are the advantages and disadvantages of pharmacological, psychological and social interventions for managing common mental health problems?
- How might the evidence base for current treatments/interventions be biased?
- What types of interventions might be more appropriate for addressing common mental health problems in lower socioeconomic groups?

Further reading and resources

For screening

Whooley questions:

- During the past month, have you often been bothered by feeling down, depressed or hopeless?
- During the last month, have you often been bothered by having little interest or pleasure in doing things?

For holistic assessment

Tools to promote more holistic assessment of underlying problems contributing to stress and depression are limited, but the Wheel of Life approach (see Figure 8.2) could offer some guiding principles for assessing life domains.

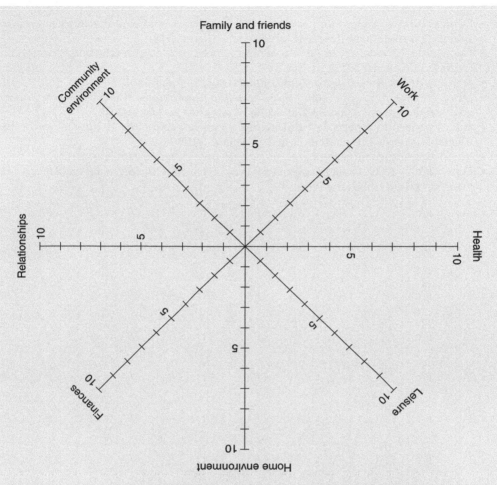

Figure 8.2 Example of a Wheel of Life Tool. Life domains are illustrative examples and can equally be identified by the individual. Life domains are then rated on a scale of 0–10, 0 representing 'totally dissatisfied' in the life domain and 10 representing 'completely satisfied'

For lifestyle management

The book, *Help Yourself to Better Health* (NHS Ayrshire and Arran 2005, see below) is full of practical advice and checklists for readers to look at their own lifestyle, and discover how some straightforward changes to their lifestyle can have a positive effect on their mental health.

General

- Clinical Knowledge Summaries: Depression: http://www.cks.nhs.uk/depression# (accessed 24 August 2012).

- Depression screening tools: www.patient.co.uk/doctor/Recognising-and-Screening-for-Depression-in-Primary-Care.htm (accessed 24 August 2012).
- Depression screening tools: www.fpnotebook.com/psych/exam/DprsnScrngTls.htm (accessed 24 August 2012).
- Steps for Stress: www.glasgowsteps.com (accessed 24 August 2012).
- NHS Ayrshire and Arran (2005) *Help Yourself to Better Health*. Available at www.scotland.gov.uk/Publications/2006/03/22091556/17 (accessed 24 August 2012)
- Computerized/Internet-based and free to access self-help CBT: Living Life to the Full. Available at www.llttf.com/ (accessed 24 August 2012).
- MoodGym: http://moodgym.anu.edu.au/welcome (accessed 24 August 2012).
- Dowrick, C. (2005) *Beyond Depression: A New Approach to Understanding and Management*. Oxford: Oxford University Press.

Part 3
Quality of life for people with mental health problems

9 Recovery and wellbeing

Mary O'Hagan

Recovery in mental health happens when a person has the personal resources, services, supports, opportunities and rights to achieve the lives they choose. Services using a recovery approach emphasize hope, self-determination, a broad choice of services and equal participation in society.

Recovery is not a new concept in mental health. Versions of it can be found in the moral treatment regimes in the early asylum era, which emphasized non-restraint, self-discipline and therapeutic optimism (Shorter 1997: 8–22; Porter 2002: 103-118) and in post-Second World War social psychiatry, which heralded therapeutic communities and community-based services (Warner 2004: 118–120). Moral treatment, social psychiatry and the current recovery movement have all been liberatory responses to coercion, poor conditions and therapeutic pessimism.

Recovery as we know it today has its origins in the user/survivor movement and psychiatric rehabilitation. The user/survivor movement began in the early 1970s, around the same time as the civil rights movement, the gay rights movement, the women's movement and indigenous movements. All these movements have in common the experience of oppression and the quest for self-determination. People diagnosed with mental illness were oppressed by institutions, forced treatment and social exclusion that condemned many to poverty, inactivity, low self-esteem, inadequate housing, isolation and exploitation. The major user/survivor movement responses were political action and alternative peer-led services (Chamberlin 1978; O'Hagan 1994).

The purpose of psychiatric rehabilitation is to help people overcome the functional limitations created by their mental illness, through individual skills development (such as social or vocational skills) and environmental management (such as social inclusion activities or working with employers) (Craig 2006; Rossler 2006). Psychiatric rehabilitation can be practised by a range of professionals delivering a combination of pharmacological treatment, independent living and social skills training, psychological support to clients and their families, housing, vocational rehabilitation, social support and network enhancement and access to leisure activities (US Department of Health and Human Services 1999).

The user/survivor movement views of recovery and the psychiatric rehabilitation views overlap considerably and some of the differences are in emphasis only. But the ownership of the versions differs and so do some of the fundamental beliefs they rest upon.

Psychiatric rehabilitation comes from a history of viewing people with lived experience largely as victims of their own pathology and the deficits that arise from it. The user/survivor movement views people as limited not so much by their individual distress, but by services and society.

At the risk of oversimplification, these two different starting points appear to generate some important differences. The user/survivor movement tends to view 'mental illness' as a social construct that can limit people's chances of recovery, whereas the psychiatric rehabilitation view tends to see mental illness as a very real condition that must be treated and rehabilitated in order for people to achieve recovery. Standard psychiatric rehabilitation is more at ease with deficits thinking, risk management and compulsory interventions, which are still a big part of today's mental health system. The user/survivor movement view suggests a more radical shift is needed, such as the demotion of pathological explanations, a greater emphasis on achieving the lives we want than in just reducing symptoms, a sizeable shift from institutions and professional experts to peer and community supports, and an emphasis on fostering personal resourcefulness.

Origins of recovery

Since the term recovery began to be used in mental health discourse in the late 1980s, the lens through which it is viewed have become progressively broader, like ripples on water. Initially recovery was mainly seen through the lens of personal experience, then it broadened to service and system responses, and later to wider social responses towards people with a diagnosis of mental illness. In recent years recovery has entered into the discourse on whole of population wellbeing.

The user/survivor movement, with its beginnings in the 1970s, critiqued medical hegemony, coercion and psychiatric pessimism. This laid the groundwork for the initial literature that used the term recovery in mental health. Patricia Deegan (1988, 1990, 1992) was the best known contributor to this early literature. She focused on the personal experience of recovery and the interactions that helped or hindered it. People do not just have to recover from mental illness but from 'the effects of internalised stigma, learned helplessness, institutionalisation, poverty, homelessness and the wounds of spirit-breaking' (Deegan 1990: 1). Recovery is finding 'a new and valued sense of self and purpose'. It is 'a process, a way of life, an attitude, and a way of approaching the day's challenges' (Deegan 1988: 15); it is not perfectly linear and it is unique to everyone. Personal recovery was clearly defined as the process of people with mental illness achieving the lives they want, whereas clinical recovery is a positive response to treatment. The early user/survivor writers on recovery laid down the challenge to mental health systems and society to help personal recovery rather than hinder it.

In 1993, a psychiatric rehabilitation expert, William Anthony wrote a guiding vision for mental health services based on the recovery concept, developments in community-based services and a broad understanding of the multiple impacts of mental illness on the individual. In order to support recovery service systems need to respond to the multiple impacts with multiple responses, such as treatment, rehabilitation, rights protection and self-help (Anthony 1993). More detailed and far-reaching attempts to describe recovery-based service systems followed, including from Anthony himself (Anthony 2000; Compagni et al. 2006; Sainsbury Centre for Mental Health 2006; Davidson et al. 2007; Future Vision Coalition 2008; Mental Health Advocacy Coalition 2008).

From the mid-1990s some new initiatives began that focused on the need for wider society to enable recovery. National programmes to counter stigma and discrimination were established, such as Like Minds, Like Mine in New Zealand and See Me in Scotland, followed by a ground-breaking conceptual exploration and critique of antidiscrimination work (Sayce 2000). Social inclusion efforts for people with a diagnosis of mental illness got underway in England (Office of the Deputy Prime Minister 2004), Australia (Australian Social Inclusion Board 2008) and elsewhere. These programmes were designed to remove attitudinal, behavioural and systemic barriers to the equal participation of people diagnosed with mental illness in their communities. By the 2000s the recovery literature was also starting to make much more explicit reference to wider societal and environmental factors in recovery (Jacobsen and Greenley 2001; O'Hagan 2001; Onken et al. 2002).

There is a good evidence base from research exploring people's views on what helps and hinders their recovery that supports the development of recovery-based service systems and the establishment of antidiscrimination and social inclusion programmes (Tooth et al. 1997; Lapsley et al. 2002; Onken et al. 2002; Mental Health Commission 2004). The following themes emerged as helpful to focus on.

- Hope is fundamental to recovery.
- Self-esteem, confidence, and getting rid of internalized stigma.
- Personal resourcefulness through learning, making choices, self-management and persistence.
- Relationships that are respectful, strengths-based, supportive and reciprocal.
- Income sufficient to cover basic living needs, housing and transport.
- Contribution through work, education or recreation.
- Transitions in life circumstances, place or cultural or personal identity.

Recovery and population wellbeing

The connection between personal recovery and a new way of delivering services is well established and documented, as is the connection between personal recovery and antidiscrimination and social inclusion programmes. The rest of this chapter makes a case for extending our recovery thinking and practice into the whole of population wellbeing agenda.

In the 2000s a critical mass of new thinking and evidence in positive psychology, happiness, wellbeing and social capital considered the rationale and methods for increasing the wellbeing of the whole population (Seligman 2002; Marmot 2004; New Economics Foundation 2004, 2008; Layard 2005; Wilkinson 2005; The Government Office for Science 2008; WHO and the Commission on Social Determinants of Health 2008, Wilkinson and Pickett 2009b). This work has improved our knowledge of wellbeing and loss of wellbeing – their determinants, consequences, and the interventions needed to increase population wellbeing.

Traditionally, mental health and mental illness have been conceptualized as two ends of a continuum that require very different responses – prevention and promotion for people at the mental health end, and services and treatments for people at the mental illness end. This approach is illustrated conceptually in the mental health intervention spectrum for mental disorders (Mrazek and Haggarty 1994) that places prevention, treatment and maintenance on a continuum with a series of interventions ranging from universal prevention for the general public to aftercare and rehabilitation for people with 'serious mental illness'. This division between promotion and prevention at one end and treatment and services at the other also has been reflected in the traditional separation of prevention and services in policy, agency structures and responsibilities, and in practice in many Western countries (O'Hagan 2006). Whole systems, organizational structures and professional groups have been built on the assumption that people at the healthy end of the spectrum have a very different set of needs to people at the illness end.

This single continuum approach has been criticized (Tudor 1996; Keyes 2002, 2007) because there is mounting evidence that the absence of mental health does not necessarily imply the presence of mental illness or vice versa; mental health and mental illness should not be placed on the same continuum but regarded as two interrelated human conditions. This is because there are people with minimal mental health or wellbeing (languishing) who do not have a diagnosable mental illness, but endure some of the same personal, social and economic consequences. Conversely, a minority of people with a diagnosable mental illness have optimal (flourishing) or moderate wellbeing; these people do about the same as people who have poor wellbeing (languishing) but do not have a diagnosable mental illness.

Those who have both a diagnosable mental illness as well as poor mental health are the worst off. Under 20 percent of the population has optimal mental health (flourishing); this group enjoys better health, more productivity, better relationships and more resilience than people with moderate or poor mental health. The risk of mental illness increases as a person's mental health decreases, but the waning of the symptoms of mental illness is, on average, associated with only a modest increase in mental health (Keyes 2002, 2007).

If we think in terms of two intersecting continua – the first being optimal wellbeing (flourishing) to minimal wellbeing (languishing), and the second being a high degree of mental illness to no mental illness, it is no longer feasible to continue to treat people with a diagnosis of mental illness as 'other' than the rest of the population. People with diagnosable mental illness cover the same wellbeing territory as people without mental illness, albeit in different proportions. A survey of Americans between the ages of 25 and 74 showed that of the people in the population with a diagnosis of mental illness, 30 in 100 have minimal wellbeing, compared with 12 people in 100 with no diagnosis of mental illness; 63 people in 100 with a diagnosis have moderate wellbeing, compared with 66 people in 100 without a diagnosis; and 7 people in 100 with a diagnosis have optimal wellbeing, compared with 22 people in 100 without a diagnosis (Keyes 2007: 103).

For people with a diagnosis personal recovery is highly associated with the movement towards optimal wellbeing on the wellbeing continuum, whereas clinical recovery is highly associated with moving towards no symptoms or mental illness diagnosis on the mental illness continuum. Personal recovery for people with a diagnosis therefore has many features in common with recovery from loss of wellbeing of any kind (Slade 2010).

In addition to the conceptual overlapping of mental illness and loss of wellbeing, there is evidence that the determinants, consequences and effective interventions for people with minimal wellbeing, with or without a diagnosable mental illness, are similar.

Wellbeing in humans has a number of determinants; our genes and upbringing; our external circumstances such as employment status, marital status and even the weather; and our own attitude to life and sense of involvement in the world (New Economics Foundation 2004). Psychosis and other serious mental illness diagnoses have been commonly viewed in psychiatry as genetically determined, but there is growing evidence that broader determinants such as trauma and inequality are associated with the development of psychotic conditions (Read et al. 2004) and not just ordinary loss of wellbeing. Developments in genetics have also highlighted the complex interrelationship between our genes and our environment (Ridley 2003). Current evidence has identified the following social determinants in the development of loss of wellbeing and mental illness.

- Trauma – abuse and neglect in early life, war, physical or sexual assault.
- Inequality – particularly relative poverty, lack of hierarchical status and racism.
- Deculturation – particularly for indigenous people.
- Oppression – subjugation, slavery, living in totalitarian states.
- Fragmented communities, extreme individualism and the loss of shared values.

(Marmot 2004; Harris et al. 2005, 2006; Wilkinson 2005; Keyes 2007; The Government Office for Science 2008; WHO and the Commission on Social Determinants of Health 2008; Wilkinson and Pickett 2009b).

The consequences of loss of wellbeing and mental illness are also similar. They are not just personal, they are social and economic too:

- less psychological resilience;
- poorer relationships;
- poorer productivity;
- poorer physical health;
- a shorter lifespan.

(Marmot 2004; Harris et al. 2005; Wilkinson 2005; Keys 2007; The Government Office for Science 2008; WHO and the Commission on Social Determinants of Health 2008; Wilkinson and Pickett 2009). People who experience just loss of wellbeing or just mental illness suffer these consequences less severely than people who experience both (Keyes 2007).

There is an emerging evidence base for government interventions designed to increase the wellbeing of the population. These are summarized in the Table 9.1.

Table 9.1 Evidence-based government interventions to improve wellbeing

Population group	Evidence-based government interventions to improve wellbeing
All citizens	Wealth redistribution through taxation Sufficient income for all, including those who cannot earn Universal healthcare that promotes health and wellbeing as well as treating illness Active citizen involvement in local communities, public services and the political process Lifelong access to education Reduction in inequality and marginalization of indigenous people and minorities
Children	Support and coaching for parents, particularly from disadvantaged groups Early intervention with childhood emotional, behavioural and learning problems Stable, healthy housing A broad education curriculum that promotes wellbeing and maximies educational attainment Restrict advertising directed at children and young people Family friendly employment policies, e.g. part-time work, flexible working hours, parental leave
Adults	Stimulate the demand for skills Empower people to learn and to fill skill shortages Uphold fair employment laws Promote mentally healthy workplaces with focus on wellbeing and work/life balance
Older adults	Encourage social and educational opportunities and networks Encourage work and productivity in older people Address the stigma and discrimination associated with old age
People with a diagnosis of mental illness	Address the link between debt and mental illness Provide access to wellbeing promotion Ensure access to a broad range of therapeutic and support services Provide support for employment Address stigma and discrimination

Sources: Durie 2004; New Economics Foundation 2004, 2008; Harris et al. 2005; Layard 2005; Wilkinson 2005; Harris et al. 2006; Keyes 2007; McDaid et al. 2007; The Government Office for Science 2008; WHO and the Commission on Social Determinants of Health 2008; Wilkinson and Pickett 2009b.

All the above evidence-based interventions for the whole population and different age groups will also benefit people with a diagnosable mental illness and they may be enough on their own to help move people with mental illness to the more favourable end of both continua. If not, people with mental illness will need the specific interventions indicated in the last row of the table.

The two continua model breaks down the long-held conceptual and practice divide between people with mental illness and people without it. The similarities in the determinants, consequences and interventions for people with both loss of wellbeing and mental illness suggests that we need to consider these two sometimes overlapping groups as a whole with subsets, rather than two separate categories. The recovery approach in mental health, with its emphasis on increasing wellbeing rather than just decreasing mental illness, also helps to breakdown the division between people with a diagnosable mental illness and people without it. The integration of recovery and whole of population wellbeing needs to happen at the legislation and policy level, in funding and delivery and in research. This requires government ministries, departments and agencies to cooperate and integrate much more with each other, and also with the third sector and the business community (McDaid et al. 2007; Raeburn 2008; The Government Office for Science 2008; WHO and the Commission on Social Determinants of Health 2008).

There is more than just an inevitable logic to integrating mental health recovery into whole of population wellbeing. It also has several implications for the fairer distribution of power and resources. Combining recovery with whole of population wellbeing may weaken the medical dominance and deficits approaches within the mental health system if concepts, policies and service delivery for both groups are much more integrated. In recent years some recovery pioneers in the user/survivor movement have commented that the mental health system has adopted recovery rhetoric without undergoing a deeper paradigm shift. Some no longer want to identify with the term 'recovery' (Wallcraft 2009). The broader wellbeing agenda gives us new language that cannot so easily be co-opted by a system that is still driven by medical and deficits-based approaches. Moving recovery into the whole of population wellbeing agenda also has the potential to erode stigma and discrimination because people with a diagnosis of mental illness are no longer 'other'; they share many experiences and attributes with anyone in the community who struggles with wellbeing. In the past 20 years users and survivors as well as their professional allies have developed a body of knowledge and skills relating to recovery, much of which is as relevant to people with loss of wellbeing as it is to people with a diagnosable mental illness. Moving recovery into the whole of population wellbeing agenda will make this knowledge base more available for all who could benefit from it. Finally, the combining of recovery and wellbeing could mean that more resources are made available to people with a diagnosable mental illness, because wellbeing is a whole of government responsibility, whereas recovery on its own has stayed largely a mental health sector responsibility. We are just beginning to see the potential of this integration.

Mini toolkit

Tips for effective practice: recovery and wellbeing – the destination and the pathways

This chapter has offered a broad theoretical perspective on recovery for people with a diagnosis of mental illness and its relationship to whole of population wellbeing. The purpose of this mini toolbox is to give the reader some assistance in applying this theoretical perspective in their work. We start with a destination picture of a system that fits the theoretical framework offered in this chapter (see Box 9.1).

Box 9.1 The eight-level destination: an outline of a system that supports recovery and wellbeing

This destination picture covers the whole system, from attitudes to the systemic framework.

1. *Attitudes*: to create deep transformation in services we need to change some of our fundamental beliefs, particularly the view that madness has no value or meaning. If madness is primarily seen as brain pathology, the purpose of services is to correct brain pathology through medical expertise and at times containment.
2. *Purpose*: if madness is seen as a fully human but challenging state of being with multiple determinants and consequences, the purpose of services might be for service users to lead their own recovery in a milieu that is underpinned by hope, self-determination, a broad range of responses and social inclusion.
3. *Behaviour*: the purpose of services determines everything that goes on in services from human behaviour to the systemic framework in which they operate. Recovery-based services demand changes in human behaviour. Whereas service users were once expected to be passive recipients of expert interventions, in a recovery-based service they need to be active agents and leaders in their own recovery. The people working in services are no longer expected to be 'on top', instead they need to be 'on tap'. Families need to learn how to support recovery. Communities, opinion leaders and politicians need to show zero tolerance of discrimination.
4. *Culture*: the behaviour expected of people also helps to determine the core elements of services, or their underlying culture. For instance, services that exist largely to correct brain pathology where professionals are regarded as expert authorities may favour clinical or institutional environments, objective and impersonal language, and a narrow evidence base that upholds their professional privilege. These services also have a social control function that allows the use of compulsory detention, treatment and physical force. A transformed recovery-based system will, on the other hand, favour natural non-institutional environments, value service users' subjectivity, work in partnership with service users at all levels, and minimize or eliminate compulsory interventions. A recovery-based service will have extensive community networks to draw upon instead or working in isolation.
5. *Responses for individuals*: all this leads to the responses that are actually delivered to people using services. The latest policy and evidence as well as service-user expectations, indicates we need a much broader range of services than are available to most people at the moment. Most of these responses are not medical, and few or any of them should take place in institutional or clinical settings. Service navigation, peer support, recovery education, advocacy, personal assistance in crisis and support in education, employment and housing, as well as some complementary and talking therapies, must be as available as drug therapy is now to all people who are diagnosed with mental distress or experience loss of wellbeing.
6. *Responses to populations*: the larger system is also responsible for delivery to populations. In a transformed system, prevention should no longer be confined to a branch of the health bureaucracy, but become a whole of government responsibility. Governments need to develop social and economic policy that minimizes trauma and inequality, and optimizes well-being. They need to measure well-being in the population to help them create and monitor policy. The delivery of mental health promotion should provide the awareness, information and skills for all citizens, including people diagnosed with mental illness, to maximize their well-being. Society's responses to people who have developed serious mental distress needs to be modified through comprehensive antidiscrimination and social justice programmes.

7. *Integration and coordination*: the people and agencies that serve both individuals and populations need to find new ways to work together, for example, through joint planning and pooled funding, through moving workforces between teams, services and sectors, through information sharing, or shared use of communications technologies for online or distance service provision. Many services now delivered within the specialist mental health sector could be delivered by primary health or social services, and in community organizations rather than statutory ones.

8. *Systemic framework*: a transformed mental health system needs an overarching systemic framework. Legislation that affects people with a diagnosis of mental illness and loss of wellbeing needs focus on human rights and fostering equality. Policy and funding must span across sectors and push services into the future rather than reinforcing the status quo. The development of research, the workforce and services needs to lead towards the recovery-based destination. At the local, state and national levels there needs to be well-resourced oversight of services led by the people who use them and their communities.

Finally, once we have a destination, we can start to create a coherent network of pathways to get there. We need to create pathways that offer the most leverage in relation to the human and financial resources put in. If the following pathways were created and sustained, we could reach the destination of transformed services.

This is followed by brief descriptions of the systemic pathways and human interactional pathways that lead towards the destination (see Box 9.2).

Box 9.2 Ten systemic pathways: strategies for developing a recovery and wellbeing system

Here are the ten systemic pathways in summary form.

Core services
1. Develop new core services and associated workforces – peer support, recovery education, support for independent housing, employment and education support, advocacy and talking therapies.
2. Recruit workers into services with lived experience and recovery values as well as skills; train all workers in recovery competencies, and link training to ongoing coaching and performance appraisal.
3. Replace most hospital services with services in people's homes, online or embedded in communities, and establish home- and community-based crisis services.

Human rights and equality
4. Work towards ending special mental health legislation, drastically reduce compulsory interventions and eliminate seclusion and restraint.
5. Run ongoing recovery and human-rights-based antidiscrimination and social justice campaigns, for the general public and target groups, and led by service users.
6. Advocate for a whole of government commitment to prevention and promotion through minimizing inequality and trauma, optimizing wellbeing and measuring wellbeing.

Measures and outcomes

7. Develop robust evidence and measures through service user-led and community-led participatory research and evaluation.
8. Develop targets for increasing the participation of people with serious mental health problems in the open labour market and in independent housing.

Systemic drivers

9. Develop structures, funding and incentives for intersectoral cooperation and integration in services.
10. Develop local stakeholder leadership groups, with a majority of service users and families on them, and resourced by staff – to identify the needs of their communities, monitor services across sectors, and set directions for cross-sector service development.

The systemic pathways are most relevant to people in high-level management, commissioning or policy roles. The interactional pathways are most relevant to people in direct service delivery roles and team leaders (see Box 9.3).

Box 9.3 Seven interpersonal pathways that support recovery and wellbeing

Here are the seven interpersonal pathways in summary form.

1. Communicate that mental distress is an extremely challenging but essentially human experience that value and meaning can be derived from.
2. Show hope and non-judgemental belief that people can live the lives they choose, especially when they are stuck or have setbacks.
3. Ensure full attention is given to the psychological, social, economic, spiritual and biological determinants and consequences of people's mental distress.
4. Amplify and enlist people's strengths and support them to maximize their own opportunities and manage their own risks.
5. Facilitate people to claim or reclaim full social and economic participation in their communities, recognizing they have the same needs, rights and aspirations as other citizens.
6. Support the prevention of compulsory treatment and other coercive practices.
7. Support the leadership of people with mental distress in the development, delivery and valuation of services, as individuals and as a collective.

Case studies: Recovery networks and recovery colleges

The Scottish Recovery Network (www.scottishrecovery.net) was established to raise awareness of recovery, to learn more about the recovery experience and to share ideas and encourage action to promote recovery in Scotland. SRN develops publications and resources; conducts research; supports the development of local recovery networks; supports mental health services to become more recovery oriented; and supports the development of the peer support workforce in Scotland. Some of its key projects have been narrative research into the experience of recovery, the development of learning materials for mental health workers, the promotion of Wellness Recovery Action Planning (WRAP) for people with mental illness, and the development of the Scottish Recovery Indicator for mental health services to assess their recovery orientation. Recovery Devon (www.recoverydevon.co.uk) is a local recovery network that supports recovery at the personal and service levels. Recovery colleges provide educational opportunities for people using and working in services. Their educational approach is designed to help rebuild lives rather than standard therapeutic approaches that focus upon reducing symptoms. People who participate take on the role of student rather than service user. Recovery colleges have been established in South West London (www.swlstg-tr.nhs.uk) and in Nottingham (www.nottinghamshirehealthcare.nhs.uk) and elsewhere. See Table 9.2 to see how the Scottish Recovery Network contributes.

Table 9.2 How the Scottish Recovery Network contributes to the systemic and interactional recovery pathways

Systemic pathways

Develop new core services and associated workforces – peer support, recovery education, mobile housing support, employment and education support, advocacy and talking therapies	Promotes the development of peer support and recovery education
Recruit workers into services with lived experience and recovery values as well as skills; train all workers in recovery competencies, and link training to ongoing coaching and performance appraisal	Contributes to the recovery training of Scottish mental health workers
Develop robust evidence and measures through service user-led and community-led participatory research and evaluation	The development of the Scottish Recovery Indicators and narrative research

Interactional pathways

Communicate that mental distress is an extremely challenging but essentially human experience that value and meaning can be derived from	The promotion of recovery experiences and stories
Show hope and non-judgemental confidence that people can live the lives they choose, especially when they are stuck or have setbacks	The promotion of recovery experiences and stories
Amplify and enlist people's strengths and support them to maximize their own opportunities and manage their own risks	The facilitation of wellness recovery action plan (WRAP) planning
Support the leadership of people with mental distress in the development, delivery and evaluation of services, as individuals and as a collective	The development of local recovery networks

Reflection points and questions

For people who work directly with service users

Think about your place in the world:

- the purpose of your organization;
- your role within the organization;
- your sphere of influence.

Consider the areas in which you can best support recovery and wellbeing:

- identify the destination levels most relevant to your role;
- identify the pathways most relevant to your role.

Plan how you will initiate and sustain the change you want to make:

- the rationale for the change and how you will communicate it;
- the support you need from leaders and stakeholders to make the change;
- the opportunities to be maximized – within yourself, the system you work in, and the wider world;
- the constraints to be overcome – within yourself, the system you work in, and the wider world;
- strategies for sustaining the change.

For service and system leaders

People who lead teams, services or systems can identify the contribution different people or different parts of the system make towards the recovery destination by identifying the pathways they are working on. This may also be a good way to identify where there are gaps in the total team, service or system efforts to reach the destination.

Further reading and resources

- Scottish Recovery Network: www.scottishrecovery.net (accessed 24 August 2012).
- Centre for Mental Health: www.centreformentalhealth.org.uk/recovery/index.aspx (accessed 24 August 2012).
- Recovery Devon: www.recoverydevon.co.uk/ (accessed 24 August 2012).
- Recovery Colleges: www.centreformentalhealth.org.uk/pdfs/Recovery_Colleges.pdf).
- National Empowerment Center: www.power2u.org/ (accessed 24 August 2012).
- National Coalition for Mental Health Recovery: http://ncmhr.org/ (accessed 24 August 2012).
- The Copeland Center and WRAP: www.mentalhealthrecovery.com/ (accessed 24 August 2012).
- Building a Culture of Recovery: www.cultureofrecovery.org/ (accessed 24 August 2012).

10 Stigma, discrimination and mental health

Nicolas Rüsch and Patrick W Corrigan

Introduction

Individuals with mental illness have to deal with two sets of problems. First, they have to cope with the symptoms of their illness. A second, and often more distressful burden, is stigma and discrimination, which is prevalent in societies all over the world (Angermeyer and Dietrich 2006; Thornicroft et al. 2009). Because mental illness stigma often leads to status loss and social exclusion in various life domains such as personal relationships, work, housing or access to care, it is a major public health concern. There is a rich body of research on mental illness stigma in particular (Corrigan 2005; Thornicroft 2006; Hinshaw 2007; Corrigan et al. 2011) and on the concepts of stigma and discrimination in general (Link and Phelan 2001; Major and O'Brien 2005; Nelson 2009; Dovidio and Gaertner 2010). Here we will briefly define three areas in which stigma and discrimination can operate: public stigma, self-stigma and structural discrimination. We will then discuss the impact these types of stigma have on people with mental illness. Finally, we will outline a few ongoing initiatives meant to reduce stigma and discrimination.

Types of stigma and their impact

Public stigma

Public stigma comprises reactions of the general public towards a group based on preconceptions about that group. For example, if members of the public consider people with mental illness dangerous, they will avoid them. Stigma is a broad term that is linked to the seminal work of Erving Goffman who defined it as a discrediting attribute that reduces the stigmatized person 'from a whole and usual person to a tainted, discounted one' (Goffman 1963: 3). Modern concepts distinguish several interrelated components of stigma (Link and Phelan 2001; Corrigan 2005). First, in order to become the source of stigma, a characteristic or cue, such as skin colour must be used to label individuals. The cue is not readily apparent in mental illness but often inferred by association; for example, that a person seeing a psychiatrist must be mentally ill. There is no clear boundary between mental illness and mental health and across cultures perceptions of mental illness and health vary; therefore the label of 'mental illness' is a social construct that changes over time. Second, stereotypes are associated with the labelled characteristic.

Stereotypes are beliefs that are known to most members of the population, whether they agree with them or not. Typical stereotypes about people with mental illness include violence and dangerousness, blame for their condition, incompetence, rebellious free spirits, or childlike (Wahl 1995; Corrigan 2005). Stereotypes may differ between different psychiatric disorders, for example schizophrenia is associated with danger and alcoholism with blame. Third, prejudice occurs if members of the public are familiar with negative stereotypes, also agree with them, and have negative emotional reactions as a consequence ('That's right! All people with mental illness are violent and they all scare me'). Fourth, prejudice leads to discrimination as a behavioural reaction. Anger-related prejudice may lead to withholding help or replacing healthcare with the criminal justice system. Fear leads to avoidant behaviour. For example, employers often do not want people with mental illness near them so they do not hire them. As a final component of stigma and discrimination, social, economic and political power is necessary to effectively discriminate against a stigmatized group. Stigma leads to status loss; as a consequence of labelling and stereotyping the person is placed lower in the status hierarchy (Link and Phelan 2001). People with mental illness indicate that discrimination most typically occurs in relationships with friends and families, in intimate relationships, at work or school, and in treatment settings (Pinfold et al. 2005; Thornicroft et al. 2009). There is also the issue of multiple stigma, where certain groups experience particular disadvantage in relation to gender, ethnicity, sexuality, disability, social class and age. For example, minority ethnic communities often experience structural discrimination and multiple forms of stigma, including racism and disempowerment. Such patterns of stigma and discrimination vary between and within communities and are related to conceptualizations of, and beliefs about mental health (Knifton et al. 2010).

Self-stigma or internalized stigma

Self-stigma or internalized stigma refers to the reactions of individuals who belong to a stigmatized group and turn the stigmatizing attitudes against themselves (Corrigan 2005). It is a process parallel to public stigma, starting with (negative) self-labelling and stereotypes, subsequently affecting the behaviour of the stigmatized individuals. People with mental illness are usually well aware of negative stereotypes against their group. If they agree with the stereotypes, and apply them to themselves, this results in decreased self-esteem and self-efficacy ('I have a mental illness and therefore I do not deserve good treatment and am not capable to work'). Self-stigma is associated with shame as an emotional correlate (Rüsch et al. 2006) and with reduced empowerment, seriously undermining the quality of life of people with mental illness, and their subsequent motivation to pursue life goals such as work or independent living (Corrigan et al. 2009).

Many people with mental illness try to avoid the negative consequences of labelling, stigma and discrimination by keeping their mental illness a secret. Unlike other stigmatized characteristics such as ethnicity, mental illness is usually not visible. Depending on the severity and course of their disorder, people with mental illness can therefore often decide whether or not to disclose. Secrecy is a common reaction to the threat of stigma. As noted above, discrimination is anticipated so widely that it may lead to social withdrawal when people with mental illness avoid other people who are perceived to be potentially stigmatizing. Although these coping reactions may help to avoid some experiences of discrimination, they are also associated with negative outcomes, such as demoralization and unemployment (Link et al. 1991; Rüsch et al. 2009a).

A second common consequence of secrecy and label-avoidance is that individuals with mental illness may opt not to seek care because they fear being labelled as a consequence of entering treatment (Corrigan and Rüsch 2002). There is mounting evidence that both public and self-stigma are associated with care-seeking (Rüsch et al. 2009b), including implicit attitudes to psychiatric treatments (Rüsch et al. 2009d). Stigma, therefore, contributes to poor treatment participation worldwide (Schomerus and Angermeyer 2008), which is a major public health concern (Wang et al. 2007).

Structural discrimination

Discrimination does not only result from individual attitudes or intentions. Societal rules and regulations may systematically disadvantage people with mental illness, something which is referred to as *structural discrimination* (Corrigan et al. 2004). Examples include legislation, funding decisions about research and mental health services, or health insurance policies that exclude people with mental illness from insurance coverage. For example, when making decisions about health insurance coverage, an insurance employee may discriminate against applicants with schizophrenia by following the insurance company's rules of handling applications.

An example of intentional structural discrimination is legislation that inappropriately restricts the rights of people with mental illness in areas such as voting or parenting; Jim Crow laws did this to African Americans in Southern States (Corrigan et al. 2005). Mental health funding is an example of structural discrimination that seems more unintentional. According to the WHO, mental illnesses cause about 12 per cent of all illness-related disability (disability adjusted life years (DALYs)), however only about 2 per cent of overall healthcare budgets are allocated for mental health services, indicating a dramatic lack of resources (Saxena et al. 2007). This is reflected in the view of service users in Hong Kong who saw poor quality and accessibility of mental health services as a major source of structural discrimination (Lee et al. 2006). However, there is a scarcity of research on international aspects of structural discrimination.

Implicit versus explicit stigma

Because overtly expressed stigmatizing attitudes towards people with mental illness and other minorities have become less acceptable, such biases are often expressed in more indirect, yet nevertheless harmful ways (Bodenhausen and Richeson 2010). Therefore automatically activated, implicit versus deliberately endorsed, explicit evaluations have attracted increasing attention from stigma researchers (Gawronski and Bodenhausen 2006; Wittenbrink 2007; Greenwald and Nosek 2009). This work suggests that implicit negative reactions towards persons with mental illnesses can influence particularly more subtle, non-verbal or spontaneous behaviours. Implicit reactions may be less influenced by social desirability biases than explicitly reported attitudes (Nosek 2007). Self-report measures are, by definition, limited to reactions that participants can consciously articulate, but implicit attitudes may occur out of awareness (Wilson 2002). Finally, implicit versus explicit attitudes often independently predict outcome variables, particularly in the domain of stigma (Greenwald et al. 2009). Recent research has found evidence for the role of implicit negative reactions, both in the domain of public and self-stigma (Rüsch et al. 2010a, 2010b, 2010c, 2010d).

Interventions to reduce stigma and discrimination

Public stigma

Three main strategies have been used to reduce public stigma: protest, education and contact (Corrigan and Penn 1999). Protest, by stigmatized individuals or members of the public who support them, is often applied against stigmatizing public statements, such as media reports and advertisements. Many protest interventions, for example against stigmatizing advertisements or soap operas, have successfully suppressed negative public statements and for this purpose they are clearly very useful (Wahl 1995). However, it has been argued (Corrigan and Penn 1999) that protest may not be effective for improving attitudes towards people with mental illness. Education interventions aim to diminish stigma by replacing myths and negative stereotypes with facts, and have reduced stigmatizing attitudes among members of the public. However, research on educational campaigns suggests that behaviour changes are often not evaluated, and the degree of change achieved is both limited and may fade quickly (Corrigan 2005). The third strategy is personal contact with people with mental illness, based on intergroup contact theory and an effective way to reduce prejudice against various minorities (Pettigrew and Tropp 2006). In a number of interventions in secondary schools, education and personal contact have been combined (Pinfold et al. 2003). Contact appears to be the more efficacious part of the intervention. Factors that create an advantageous environment for interpersonal contact and stigma reduction include equal status among participants, cooperative interactions, and institutional support for the contact initiative. Contact is also more likely than education to improve implicit attitudes, because pleasant and constructive contact, unlike abstract information, can strengthen automatic associations between members of the stigmatized group and positive characteristics (Rudman et al. 2001).

For both education and contact, the content of anti-stigma programmes matters. Biogenetic models of mental illness are often highlighted because viewing mental illness as a biological, mainly inherited problem, was thought to reduce shame and blame associated with it. Evidence supports this optimistic expectation in terms of reduced blame. However, focusing on biogenetic factors may increase the perception that people with mental illness are fundamentally different, increasing social distance, perceptions of mental illness as persistent, serious and dangerous, and pessimistic views about treatment outcomes (Phelan et al. 2006). Genetic models also seem to have negative consequences for people with mental illness themselves, increasing fear of other individuals with mental illness and leading to implicit self-blame (Rüsch et al. 2010b). Therefore, a message of mental illness as being 'genetic' or 'neurological' may be overly simplistic and unhelpful for reducing stigma.

Anti-stigma initiatives can take place nationally as well as locally. National campaigns often adopt a social marketing approach, whereas local initiatives usually focus on target groups. An example of a large multifaceted national campaign is *Time to Change* in England (Henderson and Thornicroft 2009). It combines mass-media advertising and local initiatives. The latter try to facilitate social contact between members of the general public and mental health service users as well as target specific groups such as medical students and teachers. Similar initiatives in other countries, for example *See Me* in Scotland (Dunion and Gordon 2005), *Like Minds, Like Mine* in New Zealand (Vaughan and Hansen 2004), or the international World Psychiatric Association anti-stigma initiative (Sartorius and Schulze 2005) have reported positive outcomes.

In summary, there is evidence for the effectiveness of anti-stigma initiatives. On a more cautious note, individual discrimination, structural discrimination and self-stigma lead to innumerable mechanisms of stigmatization. If one mechanism of discrimination is blocked or diminished through successful initiatives, other ways to discriminate may emerge (Link and Phelan 2001). Therefore, to substantially reduce discrimination, stigmatizing attitudes and behaviours of influential stakeholders need to change fundamentally.

Initiatives to reduce self-stigma and to increase empowerment

Self-stigma is not a clinical problem or somehow the fault of the person with mental illness. On the contrary, it is a consequence of unfair public discrimination. However, as long as public stigma continues, many people with mental illness will internalize stigma and therefore strategies to reduce self-stigma matter. One way to reduce self-stigma is to discuss and refute negative stereotypes in groups of people with mental illness that are run by peers or professionals, using paradigms of cognitive therapy. Research suggests that to accept stigma as fair and to hold the group of people with mental illness in low regard is associated with more negative reactions to stigma (Rüsch et al. 2009c). Therefore, efforts to reduce self-stigma should enable people with mental illness to reject stigma as unfair and to think better of themselves and their group. Psychoeducation and empowerment interventions can facilitate informed choices and shared decision-making. Narrative approaches can help people with mental illness to develop a new life-story that is less focused on their illness and deficits and more on resources and recovery (Roe et al. 2010). Further, mutual-help/peer-support groups can be a source of support and empowerment, thus decreasing self-stigma (Corrigan 2005). Another approach is to promote active participation in mental illness service provision, either through consumer-operated services, or through using advance statements that give service users more control over their treatment.

Fighting structural discrimination

Improving public attitudes and behaviours is not sufficient to fight stigma, because discrimination can persist in long-lived social and cultural rules and regulations despite the best intentions of individuals. Comprehensive anti-stigma efforts can effect structural discrimination by specifically addressing legislation, mental healthcare funding or health insurance policies that disadvantage people with mental illness. Differences between developing and developed countries should be taken into account (Rosen 2006) because structural discrimination, and initiatives to fight it, depend on legal and cultural local factors.

Recent legislation in the USA and Europe against discrimination of people with psychiatric or physical disabilities offer an example of how structural discrimination could be tackled and of the limitations of this approach. Employment equity legislation aims to reduce discrimination against people with disabilities with respect to recruitment, retention and promotion (Stuart 2006). However, the compliance of employers with the new legislation is often limited (Roulstone and Warren 2005), and for people with mental illness it can be difficult to win anti-discrimination cases in court (Allbright 2005).

Conclusions

Future anti-stigma initiatives should tackle different aspects of stigma and discrimination simultaneously. In particular, they should measure success in terms of reduced discrimination as experienced by people with mental illness. Success will depend on the continuing collaboration of many groups in society, involving people with mental illness as well as key stakeholders such as teachers, mental health professionals, faith leaders, employers, police officers and legislators. Judging from the history of the civil rights movement, a long-term collaborative effort is needed to achieve profound social change and substantially reduce mental illness stigma.

Mini toolkit

Tips for effective practice

'Strategic Stigma Change' (Corrigan 2011) is a summary of five characteristics of effective anti-stigma approaches.

1. Targeted: focusing on key groups such as employers instead of addressing stigma in the whole population.
2. Local: communities that share characteristics that can be taken into account in anti-stigma programmes.
3. Using contact between people with mental illness and the target group.
4. Credible: a person with mental illness credible to the target group, for example an employer with mental illness or an employer being part of the talk on employment-related stigma; likewise people with mental illness participating as contacts should be in recovery in order to moderately disconfirm negative stereotypes.
5. Continuous (multiple contacts over time).

Case studies

Several countries have developed anti-stigma campaigns. 'Time to Change' in England (2007–2015) aims to reduce discrimination through a high-profile social marketing and media campaign, community events to encourage contact between people with/out mental health problems, and policy work with employers (www.time-to-change.org.uk). Other campaigns in New Zealand (www.likeminds.org.nz), Scotland (www.seemescotland.org) and Ireland (www.seechange.ie) adopt similar models.

An alternative cultural approach uses arts and film. The Scottish mental health arts and film festival (www.mhfestival.com) has engaged 50,000 people using theatre, film, concerts, dance, comedy and literature. Mental health service users co-produce events and are involved in question and answer sessions. Studies indicate that arts and film increase positive attitudes about positive social contributions and recovery, by constructing shared meanings and creating emotional engagement (Quinn et al. 2011a). This model is now being used in other countries including Ireland (www.firstfortnight.com).

Undertaking research and evaluation

For stigma measures see www.stigmaandempowerment.org/resources and the comprehensive review of Link and colleagues (2004). Research should move from attitude surveys to focusing on discriminatory behaviour. Future studies should be more theory-driven, for example inspired by social-psychological models (Rüsch et al. 2009a), instead of merely offering descriptive reports. Implicit versus explicit factors should be examined and targeted in anti-stigma efforts. Emotional aspects of both stigmatizers (such as disgust) and their targets (such as shame) have been neglected (Link et al. 2004). Studies should test the effectiveness of anti-stigma interventions, especially in terms of long-term behaviour change (Thornicroft et al. 2008; Corrigan and Shapiro 2010). Service users have been underrepresented and more qualitative and quantitative work is needed to fill this gap (Rose 2001). Investigations of mental illness stigma have largely neglected the impact of structural discrimination on stigmatized individuals (Corrigan et al. 2004). Finally, we need to assess cultural factors and international similarities and differences (Thornicroft et al. 2009).

Reflection points and questions

Initiatives to reduce public stigma.

- What do we want to change: knowledge, attitudes, emotional reactions, behaviours?
- Mental illness stigma in general or stereotypes associated with a particular disorder?
- Who is the target: the general public, or specific groups, for example employers or teachers?

- How do we achieve the intended change, what is the mechanism: protest, education, contact, or a combination?
- Who runs the initiative: service users, family members, mental health professionals, government or a combination?
- When do we expect change, is it a short- or long-term initiative?
- How are we going to measure the success of the initiative, whose perspective is relevant, for example self-reported attitudes of the public or behaviour as observed by service users? How are we going to address social desirability concerns (and stigma being underestimated) when we use self-report measures or interviews?
- Do we run a local, national or international campaign? Do we want to include policies that disadvantage people with mental illness, thus including structural discrimination?

Initiatives to reduce self-stigma and increase empowerment.

- How can we increase awareness of self-stigma and associated factors (for example shame) and their impact?
- Do we want to address self-stigma as an irrational thought (for example using cognitive-behavioural approaches)?
- How can we help service users to overcome the shame often associated with having a mental illness?
- Could we increase empowerment by, for example, giving service users a more active role in their treatment (consumer-operated services), treatment in the community, supported employment programmes, participatory action research?
- What role does disclosure (coming out) of one's mental illness and its risks and benefits play for empowerment? How can friends, family, employers or mental health professionals support people with mental illness in their decision whether to disclose and, if yes, to whom and when.
- We should be careful to avoid the impression that self-stigma is somehow the fault of persons with mental illness. On the contrary, stigma is a societal injustice that affects consumers.

Further reading and resources

- See www.stigmaandempowerment.org/resources (accessed 24 August 2012).
- See www.mhfestival.com (accessed 24 August 2012).

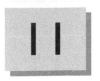

Early intervention for psychosis in the real world

Peter Byrne

One of the most resilient core beliefs in the UK, borne out by every election, survey and focus group, is the British public's devotion to its NHS. Looking at where money is spent, the cliché/truism is that the NHS is in practice a National *Illness* Service. This is especially the case in mental health services where most of our work is directed at rehabilitation, i.e. tertiary prevention – treating disorders *after* they have become well established. Medical students during their first psychiatric attachment are surprised that schizophrenia, the illness with a 1 per cent prevalence, is the diagnosis of over 90 per cent of psychiatric hospital inpatients they meet. Few of these are enduring their first admission, and frequently they have established comorbidities (depression, substance misuse, anxiety, etc.) as well as physical ill health, multiple relapses, prior multiple involuntary admissions (forced detention in hospital under mental health legislation), loss of social functioning, deteriorated family relationships, reduced social networks, non-adherence to medication and suspicion of and disengagement with services.

Early intervention

As with the best ideas, early intervention (secondary prevention) is a simple concept: intervene intensively with maximum resources at the first signs of the disorder. The interventions should be proactive and phase specific, mindful both of the developmental stage of the individual and the stage (McGorry et al. 2006) of the disorder. Since the 1970s, community mental health teams (CMHTs) knew this approach worked. Clinicians did not lack the will to intervene in young people presenting with first psychotic symptoms, and many conceded the 'system' was failing this group. In their defence, work pressures drove them back into the inpatient units, out on urgent home visits to engage or detain people with advanced illness, and into a triage role in more common presentations such as depression, severe anxiety, anorexia, suicidal acts and more. But there were other factors that prevented early intervention in the pioneering and modern day CMHTs. Twenty years ago when I started my psychiatric training, I was told to discharge patients whose psychosis appeared to be 'caused by' cannabis or 'brought on by stress'. Popular labels like 'drug induced psychosis' or 'reactive psychosis' became a barrier to following up young people likely to progress to chronic psychotic illness. This is not to deny the evidence that cannabis can precipitate an episode of psychosis in a vulnerable individual, as indeed can a stressful 'life event'. We cannot turn back the clock but these patients, now in their fifties and older, would have been far better served by the label 'first-episode psychosis', and even one dedicated CMHT member's judicious follow-up of their progress. The point here is that those individuals who made an apparent recovery should have been more rigorously followed up. In today's NHS, they are readily accepted into early intervention teams – as are patients who do not respond, the 'new long stays' in the pre-early intervention system.

The evidence base

How people present with psychotic symptoms, their evaluation, and other clinical challenges are described elsewhere (Byrne 2007), but the evidence base for the successful treatment of psychosis is worth examining (see Table 11.1). Cochrane reviews (www.cochrane.org) consistently show that the new 'atypical' antipsychotic drugs are not more effective than the older, typical agents in the longer term: the formers' side effects include less neurological problems but they have metabolic side effects such as weight gain, and promote diabetes and other hormonal abnormalities. But treating psychosis is about far more than medications, and we already have the evidence to justify innovative treatments. Old concepts such as 'therapeutic milieu' have lulled us into thinking that the very act of hospital admission is, in itself, therapeutic – but there is no evidence to definitively state that it is. It is true that people remember the need to be away from home, the support they received from nursing staff and peers, or well-run care planning meetings. But without specific treatments (Table 11.1), admission will not achieve the allevi-ation of suffering and improvement in functioning that is required here to deliver the best possible longer-term outcomes. The skills required to implement these therapies early, for example those in the first column of Table 11.1, are frequently lacking in ward staff and CMHT members. Their skill sets are about emergencies and have become almost exclusively directed towards patients with chronic schizophrenia, recurrent depression and/or personality disorder.

Without revisiting all the arguments of the opponents of early intervention, one key point was that a specialized team was not required to deliver the evidenced interventions of Table 11.1. This was supported by equivocal data that once patients received the best treatments in a timely way, the outcomes did not differ between the early intervention team compared with treatment as usual by the CMHT (Marshall et al. 2005). In short, could a properly resourced CMHT achieve as many gains in key outcomes as a specialist early intervention team? There might be parallels with assertive outreach teams, where evidence supports the assertion that a modern home treatment team does not deliver better outcomes than a properly resourced extended hours CMHT (Killaspy et al. 2006). Setting up early intervention teams is expensive

Table 11.1 Summary of Cochrane systematic reviews of randomized controlled trials that improve outcomes in psychosis

Strong evidence	Good evidence	Poor/no evidence
Cognitive behavioural therapy (CBT)	CBT early in the admission process	Motivational interviews for substance misuse
Family interventions	Nidotherapy: making changes to environment	Life skills training
Psychoeducation	Health living groups	Compliance therapy
Supported employment	Vocational rehabilitation	Supportive counselling
Integrated care for first-episode psychosis	Interventions targeting at the (well) community	Inpatient psychiatric admission

Adapted from Byrne 2007.

(recruitment costs, new premises, training, lag time until patients are recruited), and there are opportunity costs too: experienced, highly motivated innovators leave CMHTs in large numbers to work in novel settings, joining 'new' colleagues (see Table 11.2 in the Case Study below) with the promise of lower case loads. I recall the arguments of some managers to use a 'hub and spoke' model. This model is intended to deliver targeted interventions into CMHTs by skilled therapists. In reality, patients with psychosis lost out to the worst of CMHT procedural paralysis and 'turf wars', generating more paper ('it would not be appropriate for me to see X letters' and 'you missed two appointments, you are discharged') than treatments.

Randomized controlled trials prove that complex care can only be provided by a specialist team that had no other distractions. This is especially true for psychological interventions (see Table 11.2 in the Case Study below). Bechdolf et al. (2012) define 'integrated psychological interventions' as individual CBT, group skills training, cognitive remediation and psycho-educational multifamily work. When these *integrated* interventions are used in people with 'high risk mental states' (a group that progress to first-episode psychosis, often with a pre-psychosis prodrome), these patients are significantly less likely to progress to illness compared with a group of identical patients who receive (generic) supportive counselling (Bechdolf et al. 2012).

The influence of Patrick McGorry

It would be impossible to document the early intervention psychosis movement without acknowledging the individual contribution of Professor Patrick McGorry. He was highly critical of the therapeutic nihilism that mental health professionals acquired about schizophrenia, and challenged the primacy of the 'dementia praecox' concept (McGorry et al. 2005). This concept was rooted firmly in the premedications asylum era where clinicians expected to document the inevitable, untreatable, global cognitive decline in most young people who presented with psychosis. Would, he argued, cancer specialists decide that leukaemia (as a disease) is adequately defined only by children presenting with Stage 4 leukaemia? Leukaemia is a curable childhood illness, and achieving its remission – without harming patients with its treatment – is a useful parallel with first-episode psychosis (McGorry 2005). Not without irony, he highlighted that professional pessimism about psychosis outcome fuelled the anti-psychiatry movement, whereas early intervention advocates were criticized by pessimistic clinicians for their excess optimism. He also acknowledged the importance of stigma reduction through improved community awareness and other public health strategies, with the key drivers of a social movement (to promote early intervention nationally and internationally) and research (Bertolote and McGorry 2005). The case study below reflects our experience in England. The way English policy developed owes much to McGorry's principles – in particular setting out specific, essential interventions that every early intervention team needed to deliver (Department of Health 2001c). From the other perspective, early intervention enthusiasts should not promise too much in a proportion of first presentation patients. We know that the hardest symptoms to treat are the negative symptoms of schizophrenia (withdrawal, self-neglect, abnormalities of thinking with reductions in speech, etc.) and these are also frequently associated with the poorest outcomes (Simonsen et al. 2010).

Case study: setting up early intervention services

There is a joke about a bewildered tourist who stops at the side of the road to ask for directions; he is told initially by the local that 'I wouldn't start from here'. In attempting to deliver the most effective interventions for young people with their first episodes of psychosis, none of us would want to start on an inpatient psychiatric unit. But that is where I found myself twice, starting two early intervention services in north east and then west London. Thankfully, on each occasion, I worked with two experienced psychiatric nurses, all four of whom had already earned their stripes as community psychiatric nurses. We went through the notes, in one service, electronically, of every first or second admission of people aged 18 to 35. Identifying potential cases was the easy bit. We assessed everyone to confirm the diagnosis of psychosis, and then met with the individual's team to negotiate how we might take over their care. This sounds straightforward but busy inpatient units are linked to busier community teams, and neither liked strangers 'coming in here and taking our young patients'. In essence, we needed to convince these teams that their patients would get more intensive treatments, sooner, under our system than theirs. They would not become 'delayed discharges', wait a year for psychotherapy, or 'slip through the net' due to systemic failures. We did this by focusing on the short and medium term. In west London, the offices next to ours, by coincidence rather than design, belonged to the Ealing home treatment team. We approached a number of inpatients with the welcome proposition that we would get them out of hospital now, and treat them at home. But the 'medium term' meant we needed to be ready to deliver phase-specific interventions as soon as we reached agreement with the patient and his/her family. Before we could do this both early intervention teams needed the essential skills to begin treatment (Table 11.2).

The good news is that this approach helped both early intervention teams find and engage about half of our cases. I say 'good news' because this approach won over the confidence of these young people, their friends and families and their current clinicians (on the wards and in CMHTs) who, as described above, may have been resistant to the advent of early intervention teams. This was especially the case with child and adolescent colleagues who had caseloads of teenagers with psychotic relapses. These professionals had generally negative experiences of the transition of patients into adult services: family work abandoned, medication increased (on the assumption they had applied low-dose strategies), educational goals ignored, etc. The even better news is that we acquired equal numbers of new patients from elsewhere. Once we took on these hospital-based cases, we began a dialogue with multiple professionals (child and adolescent services, GPs, home treatment teams, counsellors/psychologists/therapists, social workers, professionals based in general hospitals, and CMHTs – the gatekeepers). This dialogue was about one person's experience as an example of what our early intervention team could do. Our formal letters were factual but optimistic covering what we found and what our interventions achieved (Table 11.1). We followed up these communications with telephone calls about individuals and, within the time we had available, on-site visits to our potential referrers. Time after time, they were surprised by our approach: starting early with families, waiting before using medication, phase-specific cognitive therapy, seeing people in a coffee shop until they were willing to attend a clinic, or supporting people into training, education or work, including volunteering and part-time work. Extra and earlier referrals were mostly along the lines: 'please see and assess, this young person reminds me of X whom you took on some months ago'.

Many potential referrers are too busy to reflect on what might be happening to people who cross their paths. Prime examples of this were our local accident and emergency departments. Daily, but mostly during the hours of darkness, they recorded (on computer thankfully) the attendances of young people as 'behaving strangely' – few were diagnosed, and many left before being seen by accident and emergency staff, let alone by mental health liaison teams. The differential diagnosis here includes intoxication, withdrawal (alcohol and/or drugs), crisis (any cause), delirium (medical causes of acute confusion) and psychosis. When we traced other information about these cases, we found other bizarre presentations, incomplete assessments, treatments suggested but never completed and, invariably, distressed parents. Directly, through their GPs and other health professionals, and without breaking confidentiality through schools and colleges, we offered home or clinic appointments to these 'behaving strangely' attenders.

Table 11.2 Roles and responsibilities of early intervention and allied teams

Team member	Core skills, role within the early intervention team
Psychiatric nurse	Assessment, delivery of treatments, family liaison, promoting engagement, monitoring for medication adherence and side effects, symptoms, new developments (risks to self or others)
Psychiatrist	Assessment, prescribing, proactively looking for comorbidities, agreeing the best interventions and their timing, focusing on people who were not responding to interventions, leading on risk assessment – principally self-harm and harm to others
Family therapist	Assessment of individual and family for therapy; agreeing the pace and intensity of interventions; keeping other team members informed of the content and results of family work
Psychologist	Assessing for and delivering phase-specific cognitive behavioural therapy; helping the individual feel more control over symptoms; central role in relapse prevention planning
Support worker	To engage clients in a manner they found most acceptable: informal meetings, telephone/text/email contact; to monitor social function; linking to existing/potential social networks; organizing group outings: cinema, bowling, outdoor, etc.
Vocational rehabilitation specialist	Discussing the educational and employment goals of every person accepted to the early intervention team; key interventions are needed **after** a person is placed in work – to provide ongoing support to people to remain in work
Administrator	Supporting clinicians to keep adequate records, reliable appointments (text and phone reminders for patients and family) where the team do not duplicate/overload
Outside the team	**Examples where early intervention work with other agencies**
Inpatient staff	Important for initial contacts (see text) and relapses where admission to hospital is a last resort
Home treatment team	If the individual can be treated safely at home, the transition of visits from home treatment team to early intervention team is better than hospital to early intervention team
General hospital-based liaison mental health staff	This is the cockpit of mental health crisis assessments in every region: even a weekly list of names (see text: 'behaving strangely') will maximise referrals; important in relapses too
Addictions workers	Early intervention age group has high levels of substance misuse, but this is the best/earliest opportunity to intervene to reduce this
General practitioner	Plays the primary role in the physical healthcare of each patient; will have an intimate knowledge of health issues in other family members, and earliest records of your patient
Psychodynamic therapists	There is a high prevalence of personality disorder in people with psychosis: some benefit from long-term psychotherapy
Occupational therapist	Assessment of function, ward-based activities for inpatients including exercise, interventions to enhance living skills
Social workers	Depending on the scope of their brief, can be used as a resource – and not just to achieve involuntary admission
Housing workers	Support people to achieve and maintain adequate housing; refer homeless people who had never been assessed by mental health services, or are lost to them
Police, probation and forensic services	In one London borough, 10 per cent of male early intervention patients had a history of offending, including violence; most preceded psychosis
Teachers, schools counsellors	With the individual's and parental consent (if under 16), valuable collaborators in monitoring progress and relapses
Citizens' Advice Bureau	In these recessionary times, debt may be the first 'symptom' of someone's deteriorating social function

Frequently, alcohol and cannabis were being used as self-medication – to make psychotic symptoms less unbearable – although we know both can exacerbate psychosis symptoms. More often, even at the first assessment, we could not tell for sure which came first – the habit or the symptoms. Again, a supportive observational approach will pay dividends here. This strategy is win–win: if the individual is vulnerable to psychosis, he or she needs to be within an early intervention service, but if there are no true psychotic symptoms (see Byrne 2007) then early intervention can treat the substance issues or signpost to the most acceptable interventions.

Excluding the behaving strangely group who misused alcohol or substances, careful follow-up revealed many true cases, for example a man who confronted his immediate neighbour in the belief he was the victim of invisible probes across his bedroom wall, and became the victim of a serious assault by that neighbour. There are potential referrers other than health professionals. We know that two-thirds of homeless people have severe and enduring mental illness, and key contacts here run hostels, shelters, soup kitchens and other outreach programmes. Our teams had the lower age limit of 18, but teachers and schools counsellors are a reservoir of knowledge about students' decline in social function in their late teens. Police and probation have established channels to whom they refer for a medical opinion (Table 11.2), but contact with them is a valuable educational activity.

Future directions

On the negative side, the primary prevention of psychosis and its comorbidities has received far less clinical and research attention than the two other levels of prevention. Primary prevention is true prevention – if successful, the disorder does not fully manifest. We will not develop a vaccine for psychosis, and the conventional wisdom is that the only preventable risk factor for schizophrenia is smoking cannabis – especially before the age of 14 when the brain is more vulnerable. Reducing the toxicity of urban living (van Os et al. (2004) call this *urbanicity*, and it a powerful predictor of the development of psychosis), the adverse effects of migration and social disintegration, and the cycles of substance misuse, homelessness and violence are all cited as 'nice things to do' rather than psychosis primary prevention strategies. Lloyd-Evans et al. (2011) have carried out a systematic review of interventions to reduce the duration of untreated psychosis (DUP). Neither early intervention teams in themselves nor GP educational projects will reduce DUP, and they concluded broader public education campaigns are most likely to reduce DUP. They were impressed by public awareness campaigns in Australia and Norway's TIPs programme. These campaigns are not just about case finding: care in the community will never work if the community does not care.

Mini toolkit

Tips for effective practice

- Models matter. In the case of both teams described here, other London-based services used the same model (Department of Health 2001c), with minor adaptations. London early intervention teams met two-monthly to share experiences: none of us invented an entirely new service or thought we knew it all, and no one reinvented the wheel.

- Do not break your own rules about caseloads: early intervention patients need face-to-face time to accept a difficult diagnosis and consider the early intervention team not as surveillance but support; small caseloads preserve engagement and protect staff from losing their early intervention enthusiasm and burnout.
- Keep in touch with your referrers, no matter how few or how 'inappropriate' their referrals: work hard to clarify with them what your early intervention team does and how early detection is the best possible outcome for anyone with psychosis, a prodrome or an 'at risk mental state'.
- Engaging a young person without a diagnosis but 'behaving strangely' (see text) during a period of observation is a useful activity in itself. This is not to invoke the truism that the hardest thing to do in medicine is nothing – documenting what is happening and building relationships are both of great benefit to these individuals whether they recover full functioning or go on to develop psychotic illness.
- Early intervention psychosis teams should be flexible enough to help with other psycho-social disorders that are highly prevalent in young people: relationship problems, alcohol and substance misuse, low mood, self-harm, anxiety including social phobia.
- Duration of untreated psychosis is the key determinant of outcome: the shorter this is, the better the outcomes; most strategies that achieve lower DUP rest outside the early intervention team.
- The best 'tips' for treating early intervention psychosis, and integrating public information initiatives, come from the TIPS programme in Norway (www.tips-info.com/).
- In the real world, sometimes the humanity argument (people's lives will improve) and the evidence are not enough to win the arguments about early intervention with purchasers of services. We now have economic evaluations of early intervention psychosis teams (for example McCrone et al. 2010): early intervention costs money because it saves money.

Case study

This chapter draws upon case studies of early intervention teams.

Undertaking research and evaluation

- There is strong evidence base for early intervention, however, future research in the current economic climate should examine the cost-effectiveness of early intervention versus alternative provision.
- Local early intervention teams should evaluate clinical outcomes but also the impact on individual wellbeing and the social dimensions of people's lives, including employment, education, relationships, homelessness and social networks.

Reflection points and questions

- What are the strengths and weaknesses of having stand-alone early intervention teams rather than integrating early intervention into more generic mental health services?
- What are the most significant challenges that commissioners and practitioners can face when establishing an early intervention service?
- How can you ensure that the voice and experiences of mental health service users inform early intervention practice?
- What are the likely health and social consequences of not intervening early?

Further reading and resources

- Australian Early Psychosis Prevention and Intervention Centre (EPPIC): www.eppic.org. au (accessed 25 August 2012).
- *British Journal of Psychiatry*, 187 (Suppl 48). Supplement on Early Psychosis: A Bridge to the Future (23 articles).
- Cochrane reviews: http://www.cochrane.org/cochrane-reviews (accessed 25 August 2012).
- Kingdon, D., Turkington, D., Finn, M., Wright, J, Rathod, S., Gray, R. and Siddle, R. (2010) Cognitive therapy for schizophrenia, *Schizophrenia Research*, 117: 107.
- McCrone, P., Craig, T.K., Power, P. and Garety, P. (2010) Cost-effectiveness of an early intervention service for people with psychosis, *British Journal of Psychiatry*, 196: 377–382.
- McGorry, P. (Editor in Chief of the journal) *Early Intervention in Psychiatry*: www. blackwellpublishing.com/eip (accessed 25 August 2012).
- Mental health information: www.rcpsych.ac.uk (accessed 25 August 2012).
- van Os, V., Pedersen, C.B. and Mortensen, P.B. (2004) Confirmation of the synergy between urbanicity and familial liability in the causation of psychosis, *American Journal of Psychiatry*, 161: 2312–2314.

12 Physical health of people with long-term mental health problems

Michael Nash

Introduction

There is reliable international evidence that the physical health of mental health service users is often poor, resulting in higher prevalence rates for conditions such as diabetes (Bushe and Holt 2004), risk behaviours such as smoking (McNeill 2001) and premature death (Disability Rights Commission 2005). In the UK, government policy aims to reduce mortality from physical illness of mental health service users (Department of Health 2011a). This chapter will examine the extent of physical health problems in this vulnerable group, explore reasons for poor physical health, note the role of stigma in poor physical health and finally examine how practitioners can advocate for service users rights to healthcare.

Epidemiology of physical health issues

From a public health perspective there are two key areas of concern regarding the poor state of service user physical health. First, they have a lower life expectancy in comparison with the general population. Evidence consistently shows higher mortality rates in this vulnerable group, for example Colton and Manderscheid (2006) found that when age-adjusted death rates and years of potential life lost of public mental health clients was compared with the general population in eight US states, mental health clients lost on average between 13 to more than 30 potential years of life. Chang et al. (2011) in a London, UK case register audit found a substantially lower life expectancy of 8.0 to 14.6 and 9.8 to 17.5 life years lost respectively for men and women with severe mental illness.

Second, regarding morbidity, Dixon et al. (1999) found people with schizophrenia had higher rates of cardiovascular disease, infectious diseases and respiratory disease. The Disability Rights Commission (2005) found that women with schizophrenia are 42 per cent more likely to get breast cancer and Citrome and Vreeland (2009) state that obesity is one of the most common physical health problems in mental health. These conditions can contribute to premature death as outlined previously.

However, poor physical health not only has an impact on quality of life, it can also constitute a barrier to recovery as having two complex long-term conditions such as diabetes and schizophrenia, may reduce opportunities to find or return to work, or limit the types of work that people can take up.

What are the reasons for poor physical health?

Poor physical health among mental health service users can be partly attributed to social inequalities and lifestyle factors but is complicated by the interplay between additional risk factors. Reasons for poor physical health include the following.

- *Genetic factors*: some physical conditions are partially hereditary, for example coronary heart disease (CHD) and diabetes. Therefore, a genetic predisposition to these conditions may exist, which is why exploring family history of these conditions is an important step in assessment and screening.
- *Lifestyle factors*: as with the wider general population, people with mental health problems make unhealthy lifestyle choices such as smoking or not exercising. However, service users face a higher exposure to these risk factors, for example smoking has a prevalence of around 80 per cent in people with schizophrenia (McNeill 2001).
- *Symptoms of mental illness*: experiencing symptoms of mental illness, especially severe symptoms, can have an impact on physical health. In a severe depressive episode a person may not eat or drink adequately, which can have a negative impact on the body. Negative symptoms of schizophrenia, such as de-motivation, social withdrawal and lack of volition, may inhibit a person from engaging in physical activity, which is different from choosing to have a sedentary lifestyle.
- *Adverse drug reactions*: medications used to treat mental health problems can provoke severe adverse reactions that can impede an individual's engagement in physical activity, for example movement disorders or cardiac conditions. These adverse effects can also include severe metabolic disorders such as type 2 diabetes and obesity, making medication a 'unique' risk factor for service users. Practitioners should not conflate adverse drug reactions and symptoms of mental illness with lifestyle choices, as the former are not preferences born out of freewill, but consequences of the mental illness, or its treatment.
- *Health service related factors*: some research has explored the role of non-biomedical factors in poor physical health of service users, for example practitioners lacking appropriate skills or adequate training in physical health issues (Phelan et al. 2001; Nash 2005). Furthermore, changes to the delivery of mental health services including organizational factors such as the separation of medical and mental healthcare (Druss 2007) may have contributed to an increased exposure to risk of physical conditions where people may not only fall through the service net, but receive care that is poorly coordinated between primary or adult services and mental health services.

Inequalities and physical health

Waddell and Burton (2006: vii) state that 'employment and socio-economic status are the main drivers of social gradients in physical and mental health and mortality'. Relative poverty and social exclusion adversely affect morbidity and mortality (Wilkinson and Marmot 2003). The

ONS (2000) demonstrates that people with severe and enduring mental health problems are heavily overrepresented in the lower socioeconomic groups. Therefore people face an increased risk of developing physical conditions due to their unequal social circumstances.

Being poor can damage people's physical health in many ways. It can mean living in unsafe and unhealthy housing and environments. Many service users experience difficulties making their income last for a week (Focus 2001) leading to an increased risk of poor physical health through having less financial capacity to choose a healthy lifestyle; for example inability to buy healthy foods may mean eating cheap/fast food high in calorie, salt and fat content. This is compounded by an inequity in provision of healthcare. Tudor Hart's (1971) inverse care law is also relevant here where the availability of good medical care varies inversely with physical healthcare needs.

The primary route to climbing out of poverty is through employment. Stuart (2006) suggests that work is a major determinant of mental health and a socially integrating force and exclusion from employment creates material deprivation. Yet, evidence suggests that people with mental health problems face sustained problems with finding, gaining and keeping a job. Although 75 per cent of the general population, and 65 per cent of people with physical health problems are in employment, only 20 per cent of people with enduring mental health problems work (Social Exclusion Unit 2004; Sainsbury Centre for Mental Health 2006). Waddell and Burton (2006) suggest that there is strong evidence that unemployment is generally harmful to health yet even when people do gain employment, this is frequently in poorly paid and insecure jobs (Marwaha and Johnson 2004).

Can stigma play a role in poor physical health?

Goffman (1963) defines stigma as an attribute that is deeply discrediting, leading to a spoiling of normal identity. It is usually explored from a general population perspective, or by examining service user self-stigma. Stigmatizing attitudes or behaviours of professionals are not explored to the same extent and anti-stigma campaigns are rarely directed at healthcare practitioners. Stigma is a major barrier to recovery in mental health as it leads to negative assumptions that are prevalent in both the general population and healthcare practitioners. Sartorius (2002) suggests that the public and health professionals often have negative attitudes to people with mental illness and will behave accordingly once they are told that a person has an illness. Gray (2002) states that even mental health service users who are also health professionals report a lot of prejudice from the medical profession. The Disability Rights Commission (2005) found one of the most significant barriers to healthcare identified by respondents was the perceived negative or discriminatory attitudes of healthcare staff. Lawrence and Kisely (2010) state that there is increasing evidence that disparities in healthcare provision contribute to poor physical health outcomes suggesting healthcare provider issues, including pervasive stigma associated with mental illness, are a contributing factor to poor physical health.

The stigma process in physical health

Stigma can lead to negative attitudes that can be manifested in decision-making influenced by judgement biases – what practitioners assume rather than what may be. For example, through stigmatizing ideas people with mental health problems may be discredited as 'normal' individuals by healthcare practitioners. Practitioners may make faulty assumptions regarding mental illness, for example mental illness equates with mental incompetence (Klein and Grossman 1971). Such incompetence further undermines the stigmatized person, which may result in practitioners disbelieving reports of physical symptoms, or interpreting them as manifestations of the mental illness.

This process is diagnostic overshadowing and may lead to an invalidation of service users reports of physical symptoms and is outlined in the following example (Box 12.1).

Box 12.1 Case study

John is a 45-year-old man with anxiety disorder. He has frequent panic attacks. There is a family history of CHD. John has been smoking since he was 15 and usually smokes 40 cigarettes daily. He says this helps him cope with anxiety. He does not exercise. John begins to complain of breathlessness, chest tightness and palpitations. The nurse tells John that his symptoms are psychosomatic and advises him to do some relaxation exercises.

John's physical symptoms are automatically labelled as manifestations of mental illness, even in the face of reported symptoms, present risk factors and family history. It may well be a panic attack. However, the diagnosis of mental illness has invalidated the physical symptoms and the possibility that it is a coronary event. Another aspect of diagnostic overshadowing is that the presence of diagnostic symptoms or risk factors may be mistaken as consequences of treatment, as illustrated in the following example (Box 12.2).

Box 12.2 Case study

Mary is 24 years old and is currently experiencing a psychotic episode of eight months duration. She is taking antipsychotic medication. She complains of dry mouth and her doctor advises her to drink fluids. She complains of putting on weight and always having to go to the toilet, even at night. Nurses tell her it is because she needs to drink water for her dry mouth.

Increased thirst, increased drinking and increased urination are symptoms of diabetes. Practitioners have mistaken, or conflated, medication side effects with symptoms of diabetes. Diagnostic overshadowing may mean practitioners default to a mental illness narrative without considering a possible physical cause.

Practitioners may also exhibit negative attitudes in the form of therapeutic fatalism (Nash 2011). Here practitioners assume that it is not worthwhile trying to 'change the unchangeable'. An example would be smoking cessation not being offered as there may be a belief that service users are incapable of giving up. The same may be assumed of obesity where medication that has severe metabolic side effects leaves practitioners thinking that service users cannot effectively manage weight gain as it is an inevitable chemical effect of treatment. Therapeutic fatalism can cause inertia and de-motivate practitioners, reducing the likelihood of public health initiatives – smoking cessation or physical activity – being implemented as they think they will fail.

Stigma in action?

Research shows that mental health service users often do not receive tests for assessing metabolic risk factors, even for factors that are relatively simple and easy to measure. De Hert et al. (2011) highlight how people with schizophrenia are not being adequately screened and treated for dyslipidaemia (high cholesterol levels) (up to 88 per cent untreated) and hypertension (high blood pressure) (up to 62 per cent untreated).

Two studies relating to diabetes show healthcare disparities in action. Nasrallah et al. (2006) found a low treatment rate for diabetes mellitus, with only 45.3 per cent of service users with clinical diabetes receiving any diabetic treatment. Frayne et al. (2005) found a similar healthcare disparity where people were not receiving appropriate diabetes care, for example HbA1c testing (a form of blood glucose monitoring that is important in assessing control of diabetes), cholesterol testing or eye examinations.

Why do such disparities exist? One has to assume that there is not a conscious intention by professionals to treat mental health service users with physical conditions differently than the general population. Non-treatment of identified conditions, or lack of appropriate screening in the face of huge evidence, is a major public health challenge and priority for health services and practitioners.

Institutionalized stigma?

People, by virtue of having a psychiatric diagnosis, can experience institutionalized stigma and discrimination to the detriment of their physical health. By developing a theme of institutionalized stigma we do not seek to excuse discriminating behaviour by individuals, rather try to explain it and then move to rectify it. Therefore, although physical health may be poor for a number of reasons, one of those reasons should not be due to stigma or associated negative attitudes of practitioners. This idea may be an extension of Sartorius's (2002) notion of iatrogenic stigma. Here poor physical health arises as a consequence of negative assumptions and stereotyping associated with mental illness and its stigma. These tend to influence clinical decisions in favour of practitioner assumptions rather than available evidence.

Tackling institutionalized stigma

The irony of mental health service users poor physical health is that many are in regular contact with health and social care professionals, yet common physical conditions remain undetected. In fact they often remain undetected until a critical event occurs. Even in primary care settings conditions like CHD and type 2 diabetes may go undetected.

Tackling institutionalized stigma requires an acknowledgement that there is a problem in the first instance. There may be a reticence on the behalf of healthcare professionals to acknowledge that problems with stigma exist. However, the propensity to maintain faulty assumptions about physical health must be challenged.

At an individual and organizational level, practical steps include the introduction of public health initiatives that are routinely employed with the general population – breast and testicular screening, smoking cessation, cholesterol screening and statin treatment. Clinical guidelines for managing physical conditions, for example National Service Frameworks and those of NICE for cancer, diabetes and CHD, to name a few, should be implemented in mental health settings when and where required.

Practitioners can also be active advocates for the rights of service users to physical care. They should be willing to act in an interprofessional way and negotiate with physical care providers to ensure they get timely treatment. However, practitioners may also need recourse to legal frameworks such as using disability discrimination legislation if people are being denied their right to treatment.

At management level a transformation in the way in which physical health services are commissioned between mental health and primary care services is required so that the 'who/ what conundrum' can be resolved; who should provide what, who is responsible for what, but most significantly who pays for what. However, physical health is too important to be left to statutory health services; it is an issue of social justice. Mental health organizations have much to contribute to this debate. The reality of poor physical health betrays much of the policy and management rhetoric regarding service user input and high-quality care. User organizations would be ideal partners in advocating for rights to healthcare, but also empowering service users to take charge of their own physical health. This would also be a double-edged sword, serving to challenge negative attitudes and stigma.

Mini toolkit

Top tips for effective practice

- Practitioners should routinely engage in critical reflection of their decision-making processes so that they do not conflate physical symptoms with symptoms of mental illness. This means taking all reports of physical symptoms seriously. When practitioners reflect on their own attitudes and potential biases they may be less inclined to default to a mental health narrative when service users relate physical symptoms.
- Closer interprofessional working will enhance the quality of physical healthcare provision for service users. Practitioners should develop effective outreach with local primary care services so that service users have access to services provided for the general practice population, for example well man or well women clinics. Having a model of shared physical care between primary care and mental health services would enable people to have needs more appropriately met. For instance, dual, complex long-term conditions registers could be developed as frameworks for care provision, for example a register for service users with diabetes and severe mental illness.
- Collaborate with mental health organizations in public health initiatives such as healthy eating or physical activity promotional drives.
- Ensure that evaluations are based upon clear theory of change and that service users are meaningfully involved in all aspects of research and evaluation of programmes.

Case study

Please refer to Boxes 12.1 and 12.2 above.

Undertaking research and evaluation

- Commissioners and research funding bodies should fund long-term evaluations in this area recognizing that addressing chronic physical health problems can require robust longitudinal studies.
- Studies that seek to understand the complex links between physical health, mental illness and mental wellbeing may be challenging but valuable.

Reflection points and questions

- What type of skills training do you feel you need to facilitate mental health service user physical health and wellbeing?

- What programmes could be developed to address stigma and discrimination within healthcare settings?
- How can you effectively advocate for good physical care with those affected by stigmatizing views of healthcare practitioners?
- How can you empower service users to make more positive lifestyle choices?

Further reading and resources

- Rethink Mental Health Charity has lots of information on physical health and mental illness: www.rethink.org (accessed 25 August 2012).
- The National Institute for Health and Clinical Excellence has a range of clinical guidelines that are useful resources: www.nice.org.uk/ (accessed 25 August 2012).

Part 4
Bringing it all together across the life-course

Part 4
Bringing it all together
across the life-course

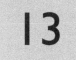

13 Parenting during the first two years and public mental health

Jane Barlow

Introduction

The parenting a child receives during the first two years of life is a significant predictor of attachment security, which is strongly associated with later wellbeing, and in particular with mental health because it facilitates the child's capacity for 'affect regulation'. Public health interventions that are aimed at promoting secure infant attachment through their impact directly on the parent–infant relationship, or indirectly on parental functioning and wellbeing, therefore provide a key opportunity for advanced industrial societies such as the UK, to promote public mental health.

The first part of the chapter examines what is meant by 'attachment' and its function in terms of facilitating the child's later capacity for 'affect regulation'. This section also examines the prevalence of different types of attachment status (i.e. 'secure' versus 'insecure' or 'disorganized'), the types of parenting that are associated with the different attachment patterns, and evidence about what the long-term consequences are in terms of the child's later mental health. The second part of the chapter presents evidence about innovative public mental health interventions aimed at helping parents to provide the type of sensitive and attuned parenting that is associated with secure infant attachment, or that are aimed at preventing insecure and disorganized attachment. The chapter will examine evidence regarding both universal and targeted interventions, alongside a number of approaches that are directed at either the parent, or the parent and infant together (i.e. dyadic interventions). The chapter concludes with a toolbox for practitioners.

The role of the early parent–infant relationship and public mental health

Attachment security – what is it and what is its function?

John Bowlby very famously identified an important developmental point in the first year of life, which he called attachment (for example Bowlby 1969, 1973, 1979). Attachment refers to the affective bond between infant and caregiver, and after many years of research, it is now recognized to be the mechanism by which the dyadic regulation of emotion takes place (for example Sroufe 1996; Schore 2001). This involves the mother (or primary caregiver) regulating the infants rapidly changing emotional states, thereby allowing the infant to develop coherent responses to the occurrence of stress (Schore 2001: 14).

Infants who are securely attached are able to use their parent at times of stress to help regulate themselves, and as a 'secure base' from which to explore the world (see Howe 2010, Shemmings and Shemmings 2011 for summaries). Attachment relationships with primary caregivers are significant because they are 'internalized' in the form of 'internal working models', which are largely unconscious representational models of 'self' and 'self with other', and are important because they provide the child with prototypes for later relations that continue into adulthood. Evidence from a number of longitudinal studies show stability for these attachment categories across the first 19 years of life, suggesting support for the view that such internal working models are stable over time (Main and Hesse 1990; Fraley 2002). Adult attachment categories have been developed that correspond with these childhood categories (see for example, Fraley and Waller 1998), and perhaps most importantly in terms of the concerns of public mental health, research shows that parental attachment status is one of the key predictors of child attachment security (Main and Hesse 1990; van Ijzendoorn et al. 1999).

The function of attachment in helping the infant to modulate affect arousal is indicated by research from the fields of developmental psychology and neuroscience, which shows that attachment security mediates the impact of the early environment on the right hemisphere of the infant's brain, and influences the rapidly developing limbic and autonomic nervous systems, the latter setting the thermostat for the child's later stress response (see Glaser 2000; Schore 2001 for summaries of this evidence).

Who is securely attached?

The research suggests that the four basic attachment behaviours (proximity seeking; secure base effect; safe haven; and separation protest) are present in most cultures, and that typically around 60 per cent of children have a 'secure' attachment to at least one primary caregiver. Around 40 per cent of infants are not securely attached to a primary caregiver, and are classified as having one of two types of insecure attachment being either 'avoidant' (25 per cent) or 'anxious-ambivalent' (around 11 per cent), with around 4 per cent being unclassified (Hazan and Shaver 1987), although these figures vary across cultures (van Ijzendoor and Sagi 1999).

The discovery of a 'disorganized' category of classification in the 1980s identified a group of children who under certain circumstances show evidence of disorganization in their attachment behaviour (Main and Solomon 1986). Disorganized attachment is characterized by contradictory or conflicted behaviour in terms of the child's approach to the attachment figure following separation. So for example, the child approaches the parent but with the head averted or with fearful expressions, oblique approaches or disoriented behaviours such as dazed or trance-like expressions, or freezing of all movement (Lyons-Ruth et al. 2005). This type of disorganized behaviour is only visible for short periods of time after which it resolves to one of the above types of insecure (or sometimes secure) organization. A number of longitudinal studies and reviews of the evidence, suggest that such disorganized attachment manifests as one of two types of controlling behaviour as the child gets older (for example van Ijzendoorn et al. 1999; Lieberman and Amaya-Jackson 2005), with some children showing signs of 'punitive' controlling behaviours and others showing signs of 'caregiving' controlling behaviours.

Up to 80 per cent of children experiencing severely emotionally abusive and neglectful parenting show signs of a 'disorganized' attachment, but it is also found in up to 19 per cent of population samples (van Ijzendoorn et al. 1999) and as such occurs outside the context of abuse (Lyons-Ruth et al. 2005).

Implications of attachment for later mental health

There is now exensive evidence concerning the long-term benefits of 'secure' attachment, and also the long-term outcomes for children who are either 'insecurely' attached, or who have a 'disorganized' attachment.

Longitudinal studies show that secure attachment in infancy is associated with optimal later functioning across a range of domains including scholastic, emotional, social and behavioural adjustment, as well as peer-rated social status (for example Granot and Mayseless 2001; Sroufe 2005; Berlin et al. 2008).

Insecure attachment patterns on the other hand appear to be associated with an increased risk of compromised functioning across a range of domains. Findings from a recent review of the evidence found that insecure attachment can interfere with peer relations, intimacy, caregiving and caretaking, sexual functioning, conflict resolution, and are associated with increased relational aggression (Lecce 2008). For example, attachment anxiety was related to negative affectivity, lack of emotional clarity, non-acceptance of emotional responses, and limited access to emotional regulation strategies. Attachment avoidance was similarly related to lack of emotional awareness, lack of emotional clarity, non-acceptance of emotional responses, and limited access to emotion regulation strategies and subjective wellbeing (Lecce 2008).

The above study found that adult attachment influences adult subjective wellbeing via the mediating influence of emotional processing and regulation, and confirmed earlier research, which showed that insecurely attached adults (i.e. avoidant or anxious-ambivalent) tended to endorse more irrational beliefs about their relationships than adults with a secure attachment style (Lecce 2008), and that this was related to diminished relationship satisfaction (see also Stackert and Bursik 2003). Research on wellbeing in elderly people found emotional support had a bigger impact on individuals with better attachment security (Merz and Consedine 2009).

However, the research suggests that 'disorganized' attachment in infancy is the strongest predictor of poor outcomes, with evidence of a clear association with wide-ranging problems in later childhood including compulsive coercive/caregiving behaviours, social and cognitive difficulties, and a range of aspects of severe psychopathology, including personality disorder (Green and Goldwyn 2002). Many of the problems associated with disorganized attachment relate to a severely compromised ability to establish long-term trusting relationships, and this reflects the early parenting of these children, in which the caregiver is experienced as frightened and frightening, and as being the source of comfort but also source of distress (Jacobvitz et al. 1997; Lyons-Ruth et al. 2005). These children develop internal working models in which the 'self' is represented as unlovable, unworthy, and capable of causing others to become angry, violent and uncaring, and other people are represented as frightening, dangerous and unavailable. The child's predominant feelings are of fear and anger, and such children are not able to use their parent as a secure base, and have little time for exploration or social learning (see Sheppings and Sheppings 2011 for an overview).

What sort of parenting influences attachment?

Attachment plays a central role in facilitating the infant's later capacity for affect (emotional) regulation, and the antecedants of attachment security involve parent–infant interaction that recognizes, reflects and helps to modify the infant's states of emotional arousal. Research focusing on the antecedants of attachment security found modest correlations for 'maternal sensitivity' (De Wolff and van Ijzendoorn 1997), prompting a search for more specific predictive factors. Recent research has focused on 1) the specific nature of the attunement or contingency between parent and infant; 2) the parent's capacity for what has been termed 'reflective function'.

Parent–infant attunement/contingency

One of the key functions of attachment is the 'dyadic regulation of emotion', in which the primary caregiver helps the infant to regulate their emotional states. Research from a numbers of disciplines has resulted in an increasing consensus that such dyadic regulation takes place in repeated moments of 'affect synchrony' in which the parent and baby are emotionally attuned, and that is facilitated by parents who are able to repair ruptures that occur following dyadic misattunement. The following quotation provides a good example of this process:

Attuned mutual co-ordination between mother and infant occurs when the infant's squeal of delight is matched by the mother's excited clapping and sparkling eyes. The baby then becomes over-stimulated, arches its back and looks away from the mother. A disruption has occurred and there is a mis-co-ordination: the mother, still excited, is leaning forward, while the baby, now serious, pulls away. However, the mother then picks up the cue and begins the repair: she stops laughing and, with a little sigh, quietens down. The baby comes back and makes eye contact again. Mother and baby gently smile. They are back in sync again, in attunement with each other. (Walker 2008: 6)

The above quotation describes the way in which sensitive parents are able to be 'attuned' to their infant's emotional states, and to react contingently. Recent research using measures of parent–infant contingency at four months showed that secure attachment at 12 months was associated with what was described as a 'midrange' of contingency (Beebe et al. 2010). This refers to parent–infant interaction that is characterized by regular episodes of the parent and infant being in synchrony, followed by disruption and then by repair. Parent–infant 'contingency' that is outside the midrange is characterized by 'interactive vigilance' at one end of the spectrum (i.e. excessive monitoring) and withdrawal or inhibition at the other end (i.e. preoccupation with self-regulation at the expense of interactive sensitivity) (Beebe et al. 2010: 87). Recent research suggests these particular forms of disturbance of turn-taking are linked to specific forms of insecure attachment at one year. For example, higher contingency was associated with disorganized and anxious-resistant attachment and lower contingency was associated with avoidant attachment (Beebe et al. 2010).

Parental reflective function

Another body of research shows a strong association between parental 'reflective function' and infant attachment security. Reflective function refers to the parent's capacity to understand the infant's behaviour in terms of internal feeling states. This body of theory suggests that the child's developing capacity for self-organization is dependent on the caregiver's ability to communicate understanding of the child's intentional stance via 'marked mirroring' (Gergely and Watson 1996). Marked mirroring refers to the way in which a parent shows a contingent response to an infant such as looking sad when the baby is crying. When parents mirror the emotion, babies are helped to recognize that their feelings are understood. 'Marked mirroring' refers to the way in which parents reflect a modified or exaggerated facial expression, which indicates to the baby that his/her distress is not the parent's distress, and can be understood and contained by them (Gergely and Watson 1996).

Research shows that reflective function is strongly associated with maternal parenting behaviours such as flexibility and responsiveness, and the use of mothers as a secure base, and that low maternal reflective function is associated with emotionally unresponsive maternal behaviours such as withdrawal, hositility and intrusiveness (Grienenberger et al. 2001; Slade et al. 2001). Reflective function during pregnancy predicts infant attachment security at 12 months, children's ability to understand other minds (Theory of Mind) skills at five years and scholastic self-esteem at 12 years of age (Steele and Steele 2008). Research also shows a significant association between parent 'mind-mindedness' (i.e. the parent's capacity to accurely interpret what their child is thinking/feeling) and later development including attachment security at 12 months (Meins et al. 2001).

Parenting programmes aimed at increasing the parent's capacity for reflective function (known as mentalization-based parenting programmes) in high-risk populations (for example substance-misusing parents) found improved maternal caregiving and infant regulation at 24 and 36 months (for example Suchman et al. 2008, 2010).

'Atypical' parenting behaviours and 'disorganized' attachment

Recent research on disorganized attachment has highlighted the important of what has been termed 'atypical' parenting behaviours. These include a range of parenting practices including affective communication errors (for example mother positive while infant distressed), disorientation (frightened expression or sudden complete loss of affect), and negative-intrusive behaviours (mocking or pulling infant's body) (Lyons-Ruth et al. 2005). A systematic review (i.e. a meta-analysis) of 12 studies found a strong association between disorganized attachment at 12–18 months and parenting behaviours characterized as 'anomalous' (i.e. frightening, threatening, looming), dissociative (haunted voice; deferential/timid) or disrupted (failure to repair, lack of response, insensitive/communication error) (Madigan et al. 2006).

The above research points to the potential importance of promoting secure attachment and preventing disorganized attachment. This requires the provision of a range of interventions that not only focus on improving the early parent–infant relationship (i.e. parenting support) but that also provides parent support, particularly to parents experiencing problems that may interfere with the parent–infant relationship (such as mental health problems, domestic violence, alcohol/substance misuse).

Innovative public mental health interventions during the early years

Possibly one of the best public mental health policy documents in terms of the provision of a range of both population-based and targeted ways of supporting secure attachment is the Healthy Child Programme (HCP) (Department of Health 2009). The HCP was recently updated (Barlow et al. 2009), and recommends the use of a range of population (i.e. universal), targeted and indicated strategies aimed at improving both the parent–infant relationship, and parental wellbeing, as part of a model of progressive universalism.

The core population-based approach recommended by the HCP is the use of ante- and post-natal promotional interviews.[1] These consist of an hour-long semi-structured interview at around 28 weeks antenatal, and then again at around six to eight weeks postnatal. It is conducted by the same practitioner, and is aimed at promoting maternal mental health and the developing relationship with the infant, and identifying the need for additional support. For example, research suggests that attachment to the foetus during pregnancy is associated with later attachment security (Benoit et al. 1997), and the antenatal promotional interview explores the mother's relationship with the baby *in utero*, and encourages positive mental representations. Where the mother appears 'disengaged' or to have very negative mental representations about the infant, this interview can be used to intervene or to provide the mother with opportunities to begin bonding with the baby. The antenatal promotional interview can also be used to identify women who are experiencing chronic anxiety/depression, and to provide them with additional psychological support. The postnatal interview is similarly used to support the provision of sensitive and attuned parent–infant interaction, and to identify parents in need of additional help.

The HCP recommends that both parents should be introduced to the 'social baby' during the immediate postnatal period, and that this should involve the delivery of information about the sensory and perceptual capabilities of their baby using some of the many media-based (for example *The Social Baby* book/video (Murray and Andrews 2005) or *Baby Express* newsletters: www.babiesexpress.net) or other validated tools (for example Brazelton: www.brazelton.co.uk or Nursing Child Assessment Satellite Training (NCAST): www.ncast.org) that are available. The HCP also recommends that practitioners promote closeness, and sensitive/attuned parenting, by encouraging parents to provide skin-to-skin care and the use of soft baby carriers, and by ensuring that parents are invited to attend an infant massage class (see Barlow et al. 2010 for an overview of the evidence).

The HCP recommends that practitioners use routine contacts with families as key opportunities to observe and support the developing parent–infant relationship. The aim of such observation is to identify the type of 'passive' or 'intrusive' parent–infant interaction in need of further support from the health visitor, or that is seriously suboptimal and requires referral to a specialist practitioner (see below for further detail) including child protection services.

Anticipatory guidance is preventive in nature and is also recommended by the HCP. Help to establish regular routines can be particularly important in deprived or stressed families, and can play a significant role in preventing emotional and behavioural problems. Anticipatory guidance should include practical guidance on managing crying and healthy sleep practices for example bath, book, bed routines, and *encouragement of parent–infant interaction* using a range of media-based interventions.

The research shows that the same methods of supporting mothers also work with fathers (for example infant massage; Neonatal Behavioral Assessment Scale), and the HCP recommends the delivery of father–infant/toddler groups that promote opportunities for play and guided observation. The research also shows that the most effective methods of supporting fathers involves opportunities for active participation with, or observation of, their baby/toddler; repeated opportunities for practice of new skills; and practitioners being responsive to individual paternal concerns (Magill-Evans et al. 2006). The HCP also points to the importance of addressing parental conflict.

In terms of the provision of indicated interventions, the HCP points to the need for appropriate referral on to specialist practitioners, and the importance of having appropriate infant mental health pathways in place to facilitate such referrals. Specialist parent–infant interventions aimed at promoting secure attachment and preventing disorganized attachment include individualized coaching by specially trained practitioners known as video-interaction guidance. Video-interaction guidance has been shown to produce a range of benefits (Kennedy et al. 2011) in very high-risk groups of parents including reducing disorganized attachment (Moss et al. 2011). Specialist interventions such as parent–infant psychotherapy should also be available to support parents experiencing a range of problems and in particular, where there are concerns about child attachment (Cohen et al. 1999, 2002). Parents should also be invited to evidence-based group parenting programmes such as Mellow Parenting (Puckering et al. 1994).

Mini toolkit

Tips for effective practice

A number of reviews have identified the key factors involved in the delivery of effective interventions. These point to the importance of the following.

- When selecting a programme ensure that the underpinning mechanisms needed to bring about change are clearly delineated in terms of their implications for practice, and that there is evidence about the effectiveness of the programme from rigorous studies (i.e. RCTs).
- Ensure that staff delivering the programme have been appropriately trained and that they receive ongoing supervision throughout its delivery.
- Ensure that the programme is delivered with integrity in terms of adherence to the manual.

Case study

The following case study provides an example, about how the theory and research in relation to reflective function can be applied in practice. Angie is 15 years of age and has just discovered that she is 28 weeks pregnant. Angie appears indifferent to the fact of the pregnancy, and has not thought about the baby much, or its implications for her life. She has not told the father of the baby that she is pregnant, but has reluctantly shared the information with her mother, who was also a teenage parent. Angie has a history of depression throughout her childhood and appears to have few friends and little social life. Angie's midwife is concerned about her and the baby, and meets with the health visitor to discuss what can be done. They agree a plan of action that is focused on: (1) addressing Angie's antenatal depression; (2) helping her to begin to 'mentalize' about this baby before he/she is born; (3) reducing her social isolation. They begin by using the ante- and postnatal promotional interviews in order to build up a trusting relationship with Angie and to work in partnership with her, to address some of the above concerns. The midwife takes her to a group for pregnant and delivered teenage parents at the Children's Centre, and links her in with one of the other teenage mothers who has indicated a willingness to act as a peer supporter to other pregnant teenage mothers. Together, the midwife and peer supporter begin to help Angie to think about this baby, and to plan for his/her arrival.

Undertaking research and evaluation

One of the best methods practitioners can use to assess whether the intervention they are delivering has '*made a difference*' is to undertake a 'service evaluation'. Whether a programme has made a difference is usually assessed in terms of quantitative assessments of the impact of an intervention on a parent. It is, of course, useful to assess parents' views about the usefulness of the programme, and what they liked/disliked, but such an approach does not provide a quantitative assessment of impact. This can be done by practitioners assessing parental and child functioning before the intervention and then again after it, and should be undertaken using some of the widely available standardized tools.

These tools can be used by practitioners in two ways. First, they can be used with individual parents to explore what their needs are before the intervention, and how much this has improved after the intervention, and what further input might be needed. Second, they can be used to assess the overall impact of the intervention by combining the scores from all parents attending the programme pre- and post-intervention, and seeing what the average change has been, for all parents over time.

The most important aspects of a service evaluation are (1) that it focuses explicitly on the aspects of parental and infant functioning that the *intervention is aimed at impacting*. An intervention typically targets more than one outcome and all outcomes should where possible be measured; (2) that the 'right' tool is used to achieve this.

Reflection points and questions

The promotion of public mental health must begin through the support of early parenting using a range of 'population-based' and 'indicated' interventions.

- What population-based and indicated interventions are you providing that will promote public mental health by supporting the early parent–infant relationship, or improve parental mental health?
- Which groups of practitioners contribute to this; are there other practitioners that could be involved?
- Effective early parenting interventions should focus on supporting sensitive and attuned parent–infant interaction and parental reflective function. Which of the early parenting interventions that you provide explicitly target the above aspects of parenting?
- What other types of interventions/services could also be provided to improve these outcomes in (1) the population; and (2) indicated groups?
- Which members of staff need 'skilling up' to enable them to work with parents in this way?

Further reading and resources

- Parent–infant interaction using an e-learning module: www.comfortconsults.com/kipstraining.htm (accessed 27 August 2012).
- Attachment: http://aspe.hhs.gov/daltcp/reports/inatrpt.htm (accessed 27 August 2012).
- Parental reflective function: Slade, A. (2005) Parental reflective functioning: an introduction, *Attachment and Human Development*, 7: 269–281. Available at: http://clarityrising.files.wordpress.com/2011/11/slade-2005-parental-reflective-functioning-14-pgs.pdf (accessed 27 August 2012).
- Still-face experiment: www.youtube.com/watch?v=apzXGEbZht0 (accessed 27 August 2012).

Note

1. The need to begin in the antenatal period is supported by research that strongly suggests that the third trimester of pregnancy through the first 18 months postnatally represents a critical period in terms of the infant's developing brain, and that it is highly susceptible during this time to adverse environmental factors of which chronic antenatal stress/depression is just one example (Bergner et al. 2008).

14 Implementing a public mental health framework within schools

Maura A Mulloy and Mark D Weist

Introduction

Schools have emerged as key settings in which to promote mental health and to prevent and treat mental health problems. This is due to a number of reasons, including the growing prevalence of mental health problems in youth, the advantages to be gained from preventing and treating issues early, the demonstrated connection between mental health and educational outcomes, and the significant access advantages of offering mental health services in a setting where youth spend the majority of their day. Utilizing a public health framework that emphasizes collaborative partnerships between school and mental health staff, schools can provide a wide range of mental health services to reach students at all levels of need – from improving the school environment and promoting school-wide conditions that boost students' achievement and wellbeing, to broad and focused prevention programmes, to early identification and intervention strategies, to treatment for students presenting with more challenging problems.

This chapter outlines the nature and extent of mental health problems facing school-aged youth; summarizes the advantages of providing mental health services within schools; describes the international movement to instil a public health-oriented framework of promotion, prevention and intervention services within schools; provides examples of how public health and education staff can work together to develop and implement such multi-tiered initiatives; and offers suggestions for overcoming barriers and enhancing partnerships between education and mental health staff. The chapter concludes with a mini toolkit section containing reflection points and questions, a case study illustrating the application of theory, tips for developing effective practice and programmes, and recommendations on future directions for research and practice.

Nature and extent of mental health problems facing school-aged youth

Epidemiological data reveal that mental health problems are on the rise in countries around the world (World Health Organization 2005), with roughly 20 per cent of children and adolescents manifesting emotional and/or behavioural issues that have a negative impact on their functioning (Kataoka et al. 2002; American Academy of Pediatrics 2004). Moreover, the WHO estimates that approximately 50 per cent of all mental health disorders have an onset during the mid-teenage years (Kessler 2009). Failure to identify and treat mental health issues early can lead to negative developmental and academic outcomes, including attendance and behavioural issues, school drop-out, substance misuse, teen pregnancy, recurring and worsening adult disorders, and suicide (WHO 2003; Cowen 2009; Kessler 2009).

Despite the growing prevalence of mental health problems and the cost of failing to identify and intervene early (Kessler 2009), only one-third to one-sixth of youth in need access mental health services (Burns et al. 1995; Leaf et al. 2003; American Academy of Pediatrics 2004). Those of low-income and ethnic or racial minority status are more susceptible to developing mental health disorders, yet are even less likely to access or receive treatment (WHO 2005). Common barriers to accessing mental health services include: stigma related to seeking out mental health treatment, transportation issues, lack of adequate insurance, lack of awareness regarding symptoms of possible mental health issues, and an over-reliance upon overburdened primary care providers to detect and treat mental health issues (Weist 1997; Dey et al. 2004; Wedding and Mengel 2004).

Advantages of providing mental health services within schools

Schools have emerged as a logical setting to prevent and treat mental health issues among children, adolescents and youth. For the following reasons, schools are increasingly moving towards a public health-oriented expanded school mental health approach.

Improved access to mental health services

Most youth in need of mental health services access them within their schools (US Department of Health and Human Services 1999; Rones and Hoagwood 2000). School-located services reach children 'where they are' (Weist and Ghuman 2002) and reduce access issues related to stigma, transportation and missed instructional time (Adelman and Taylor 2000; Mufson et al. 2004).

Connection between mental health and academic outcomes

Pervasive evidence linking mental health and academic outcomes strengthens the case for offering a continuum of mental health services within schools. Untreated mental health issues have a detrimental impact upon academic achievement (Brown and Grumet 2009; Kessler 2009), whereas efforts to promote positive mental health are linked to improved educational outcomes (Greenberg et al. 2003a; Zins and Elias 2006).

Opportunities for collaboration between mental health and education staff

Expanded school mental health programmes allow mental health providers to work closely with educators to enhance students' educational achievement and wellbeing – whether by spearheading collaborative initiatives, consulting with school staff, participating in student support teams and committees, conducting classroom observations to assess issues and monitor progress, or helping students to practise newly learned skills in real-life settings.

Opportunities to implement a comprehensive public health approach

Schools provide a natural setting to implement a public health-oriented continuum of mental health services that address all levels of student need – from school-wide interventions to promote the wellbeing and achievement of all students, to prevention efforts aimed at high-risk students, to more intensive intervention services for students with severe or chronic mental health issues (see Weist 2005).

Worldwide movement towards adopting a public health approach in schools

Growing recognition of the integral connections between mental health and academic outcomes and the costs associated with untreated mental health problems have spurred an international movement to adopt a multi-tiered public health model of mental health service provision within schools. The public health model differs from more traditional models because of its emphasis on providing promotion and prevention services *in addition to* treatment services for more intensive needs. It also encourages collaborations within and across systems in order to promote positive outcomes. This newer model of school mental health service delivery thus reflects a larger paradigm shift occurring across public health and social science fields – away from deficit-oriented models that focus primarily on treating disorders to strengths-based models that promote positive health at both individual and system-wide levels (Weist 2005; Mills et al. 2010).

These more comprehensive or 'expanded' school mental health programmes are gaining increasing momentum related to increasing national (for example the President's New Freedom Commission Report on Mental Health 2003) and international (Weist and Rowling 2002; Rowling and Weist 2004) policy support. Within the USA, the President's New Freedom Commission Report on Mental Health (2003) and No Child Left Behind legislation (2002) contain stipulations aimed at increasing mental health promotion and prevention efforts within schools. A number of countries in Western Europe (including the UK) as well as Australia, New Zealand and Canada have implemented initiatives to strengthen mental health services within schools (for example the UK's Targeted Mental Health in Schools programme; the European Network of Health Promoting Schools; Australia's National Action Plan for Promotion, Prevention, and Early Intervention for Mental Health). These strategies emanate from a public health framework, and prioritize mental health promotion efforts for all youth as well as timely access to services for students with developed mental health problems (Rajala 2001; Mrazek and Hosman 2002; Rowling 2002; Weist and Rowling 2002).

Major movements in school mental health that embody a public health approach

There are a number of major movements around the world that emphasize and provide support for school mental health efforts based upon a public health approach. These include the following.

- The Expanded School Mental Health framework builds upon school–family–community system partnerships to deliver a full continuum of mental health promotion and intervention for students in general and special education (Weist 1997; Weist et al. 2003).
- School-based health centres employ interdisciplinary teams of primary care and mental health providers to holistically address students' physical and mental health needs (Stephan et al. 2011), and are located in over 1700 schools across 44 states and Puerto Rico (National Assembly on School-based Health Care 2006).
- The European Network of Health Promoting Schools encompasses hundreds of schools within dozens of countries, and originated out of a collaborative effort by the European Commission and the WHO to integrate health promotion efforts into schools in order to create environments that better support students' physical, mental and social health (Burgher et al. 1999).
- 'School-wide Positive Behavior Support' uses a tiered public health framework to help schools establish cultures and academic/behavioural supports that improve learning and behavioural outcomes (Sugai and Horner 2002).
- 'Social-Emotional Aspects of Learning' (SEAL) is a whole-school, comprehensive approach to promoting social and emotional skills that is currently being implemented in more than 80 per cent of primary schools in England (Humphrey et al. 2008).

The tiered public health model: promotion, prevention and intervention

As mentioned previously, public health frameworks tend to include three general levels of intervention.

- *Promotion* efforts aim to promote positive outcomes for all members of the student population (also called *universal* or *primary* approaches).
- *Prevention and early intervention* efforts aim to prevent the development of disorders among groups of high-risk students, and to identify and intervene in problems early in their development.
- *Intervention* efforts aim to address more intensive needs and to treat disorders in individual students.

The following sections summarize these approaches, and include examples of how education and mental health staff can work together to develop and deliver initiatives at each level.

Promotion approaches for all students (i.e. universal or primary)

One of the most exciting aspects of the public health approach is its emphasis on promoting the health and wellbeing of entire populations. Within schools, promotion efforts often focus on building students' competencies, strengths and resources in order to enhance the health and wellbeing of the entire student body (Barry 2001).

How mental health and education personnel can collaborate to develop and implement school-wide promotion initiatives

Promotion efforts entail school-level changes meant to improve students' wellbeing and achievement (and to decrease emotional and behavioural problems), and thus naturally encourage collaborative partnerships among public health and educational personnel within and across systems, including administrators, general educators, school mental health and primary care providers, physical education teachers, community practitioners and families (WHO 2005; Mills et al. 2010). Examples of school-wide promotion efforts include the following.

- *Enhancing resilience*: by implementing a network of protective factors within the school environment (for example caring relationships, high expectations, opportunities to exercise autonomy), schools can help students build competencies to overcome adversity and achieve greater success and wellbeing (Henderson and Milstein 2003; Mulloy 2011).
- *Improving school climate*: through working at a school-wide level to develop a more positive school climate, schools can boost students' sense of school connectedness and wellbeing, which in turn contributes to higher grades and test scores, improved attendance, lower drop-out rates, and decreased emotional and behavioural problems (Scales and Leffert 1999; Battin-Pearson et al. 2000; Bruns et al. 2004; Klem and Connell 2004).
- *Mentoring and peer support programmes*: the establishment of caring and supportive relationships between staff and students and among students has been identified as one of the most important influences in supporting students' engagement, achievement, and overall wellbeing (Blum et al. 2002; Catalano et al. 2004).
- *Integrating social and emotional learning into curricula*: comprehensive reviews of social-emotional learning programmes show a significant correlation with students' improved academic and social outcomes (Wilson et al. 2001; Zins et al. 2004). Reflective of this accumulating evidence, many schools in the USA and the UK have integrated social and emotional learning through curriculum packs (for example Social and Emotional Aspects of Learning (SEAL); positive mental attitudes; life skills training) designed to enhance social and emotional skills development.
- *Building systems of positive behavioural intervention and support*: The positive behavioural intervention and support framework uses a systems-level approach to promote positive school climate and student behaviour, and is being broadly used in schools across the USA (Sugai et al. 2000; see www.pbis.org).
- *Reducing bullying*: anti-bullying programmes often consist of school-level efforts to reduce bullying and violence, and help to create school environments characterized by a greater sense of safety and caring (Gonder and Hymes 1994) that in turn contribute to students' improved achievement and wellbeing.

Prevention approaches for higher-risk groups (i.e. selective or secondary)

Prevention approaches reflect the public health philosophy that it is better to intervene 'upstream' in order to promote health and prevent minor issues from developing into full-blown disorders or poor academic or developmental outcomes (WHO 2005). Whereas promotion efforts entail environmental-level changes to improve all student outcomes, prevention approaches are delivered to groups of high-risk students with the aim of reducing the incidence or seriousness of targeted problems such as acting out behaviours, depression, anxiety and trauma (Barry 2001).

How mental health and education personnel can collaborate to identify students for participation in prevention programmes

School mental health providers can work with educators to identify potentially at-risk students for participation in prevention groups. Possible identification methods include student support teams, informal consultations between educators and mental health staff, or more formal mental health screening processes to flag students with possible emotional, behavioural or substance use issues.

Table 14.1 Searchable electronic databases of hundreds of effective prevention programmes currently in use across the USA and Europe

Database name	Sponsoring organization	Types of prevention programmes	Website address
National Registry of Evidence-Based Programs and Practices	Substance Abuse and Mental Health Services Administration (SAMHSA), USA	Substance abuse and mental health	http://nrepp.samhsa.gov/
Safe and Sound: An Educational Leader's Guide to Evidence-Based Social and Emotional Learning Programs	Collaboration for Social and Emotional Learning (CASEL)	Comprehensive social and emotional learning programmes, as well as more narrowly focused anti-violence and drug education programmes	http://casel.org/publications/safe-and-sound-an-educational-leaders-guide-to-evidence-based-sel-programs/

As the various prevention programmes in use across the USA and Europe are too extensive to list here, Table 14.1 includes searchable electronic databases of hundreds of effective prevention programmes currently in use across the USA and Europe. For example, the National Registry of Effective Programs and Practices comprises more than 150 evidence-based programmes, including over 60 programmes designed for school implementation.

Intervention approaches for individual students (i.e. indicated or tertiary)

Public health approaches also include more intensive levels of intervention to treat severe or chronic mental health issues. These treatment-focused interventions are delivered by mental health and/or primary care providers within school, and can include individual, group and family therapy, medication, and/or referral to outside community-based services when necessary.

How mental health and education personnel can collaborate to identify students for participation in more intensive treatment-focused interventions

School mental health staff can work with educators to identify individual students in need of more intensive interventions. Sources of identification for treatment interventions can include: interdisciplinary school committees, informal consultations between mental health and education staff, and/or mental health screenings designed to identify students who manifest symptoms of various disorders.

As evidence-based and effective intervention practices are too extensive to list here, please consult the searchable electronic databases listed in Table 14.1. It should be noted that evidence-based preventions and interventions often consist of expensive manualized approaches that require infrastructure support as well as ongoing technical assistance and coaching for clinicians, and as such can be difficult to implement with fidelity in a school setting (Evans and Weist 2004; Fixsen et al. 2005). Recognition of these difficulties has sparked a critical and increasingly prominent research agenda (Evans and Weist 2004; Weist et al. 2009) as well as practice modifications to ensure easier implementation of preventions and interventions within real-life settings. These practice modifications include more flexible modular approaches as well as the identification of core elements that clinicians can choose from and implement as needed (Chorpita and Daleiden 2007).

Addressing challenges and promoting effective partnerships between educators and mental health staff

Some of the more common challenges to implementing a public health approach within schools are listed below, along with suggestions to address these barriers and to promote effective partnerships between educators and mental health professionals.

Limitations on funding and personnel

Despite the advantages to be gained from implementing expanded school mental health services that emphasize collaborative prevention and promotion, schools burdened by insufficient funding and a lack of mental health personnel often default to more traditional approaches that address only the highest-need and/or special education students (Weist 2005).

Historical lack of collaboration between education and mental health

Barriers to collaboration between education and mental health personnel include: widespread perceptions that mental health programmes are simply peripheral 'add-ons' (Staup 1999; Paternite and Chiara-Johnson 2005), turf issues arising from competing demands over limited resources (Waxman et al. 1999), lack of common language and agendas (Burke and Paternite 2007) and concerns about confidentiality that impede information-sharing (Stroul 2007).

Suggestions to address barriers and promote effective partnerships

In order to build greater school support for a comprehensive public mental health approach within schools, educators must be convinced that school mental health is not a luxury or add-on service, but rather provides a crucial foundation for effective functioning and improved academic achievement. Specifically, school mental health staff must work to build educators' awareness of the integral relationship between mental health and educational outcomes, and to increase awareness regarding how mental health and education staff can effectively work together to implement initiatives that promote positive outcomes in students' learning and wellbeing as well as help to meet accountability demands (Burke and Paternite 2007).

School mental health programmes should also emphasize the many ways they can provide support to schools taxed by the increasing mental health needs of students and insufficient school-employed mental health personnel (Foster et al. 2005). Through partnering with community agencies to deliver mental health services within schools (such as the expanded school mental health model), for example, school mental health programmes can build under-resourced schools' capacity to address students' increased needs.

School mental health personnel can also increase educator 'buy in' by building positive working relationships with educators (Rones and Hoagwood 2000; Paternite and Chiara-Johnston 2005), whether by: taking time to share in conversations, providing support for teachers in dealing with challenging students, participating in school committees, working with educators to develop collaborative school-wide initiatives, and/or developing wellness initiatives for staff.

Tips for effective practice

- *Build effective relationships and partnerships with stakeholders*. To develop effective school mental health programmes and services an early and ongoing priority should be on developing and strengthening a range of relationships. Examples of activities would include:
  - invite key stakeholders in the school and surrounding community to report on school/community needs, strengths and recommendations for school mental health services, in order to promote a 'shared agenda' (Andis et al. 2002);
  - based upon the outcomes of the needs assessment, set goals that address the specific needs of the school community. For example, outcomes of the needs assessment could include: a problem with school bullying and the need for a systematic strategy to prevent and reduce it – or – inadequate levels of school-employed mental health staff, indicating a need for greater community collaboration and/or partnerships with university graduate programmes.
- *Advance high-quality programmes and services*. A second key theme area for effective school mental health practice is to systematically focus on quality assessment and improvement. This includes assessing and improving school mental health along dimensions of hiring and supporting good staff, developing collaborative relations between educators and mental health staff, improving mental health education, enhancing referral procedures, and increasing emphasis on evidence-based practice (Ambrose et al. 2002; Weist & Ghuman, 2002). An additional priority theme for high-quality services is providing training, coaching and ongoing support for evidence-based practice, ideally using some manualized programmes, but also using a more flexible modular strategy involving cognitive-behavioural skill training in the most common core elements of clinical interventions (such as relaxation, cognitive coping, and exposure for anxiety – see Chorpita and Daleiden 2010). This more flexible approach empowers clinicians to pick and choose core practice elements that are best suited to their students' needs, and to implement them in a more flexible way that adapts to the realities of the school setting.

Case study

New Beginnings High School implemented a school-wide resilience-building approach to address the needs of its low-income, inner-city student population, while also integrating group prevention and one-on-one interventions to address students' more chronic and intensive needs (Mulloy 2011). This range of promotion, prevention and intervention efforts included the following.

- A structured extended day with afternoon enrichment activities and/or internships in order to reduce students' exposure to environmental sources of risk.
- A caring school-wide climate characterized by individualized attention and a focus on relationship-building in order to increase students' feeling of trust and school connectedness.
- High expectations for students' success and built-in supports to help students realize those expectations (for example a tutoring programme, a college preparation course).
- A school-wide focus on developing students' strengths and goal-setting capabilities in order to bolster their sense of competence and motivation.

- A school mental health programme to help students learn social-emotional skills that equip them to better understand and manage their emotions and relationships.
- One-on-one treatment interventions to address severe emotional and/or behavioural issues.

By surrounding students with the above network of protective factors, the school reduced students' exposure to risk factors and enabled them to develop key social, emotional and academic competencies that resulted in increased wellbeing and academic success.

Undertaking research and evaluation

- Whole-school approaches acknowledge the interdependence of policy and practice, and are shaped by the socioeconomic circumstances of pupils. Understanding what works in school mental health requires sophisticated and multi-level evaluations. Weist et al. (2005) developed a measure for ongoing quality assessment and improvement: the School Mental Health Quality Assessment Questionnaire (SMHQAQ), which can be downloaded for free from www.schoolmentalhealth.org
- A cycle of needs assessment, priority setting, and evaluation should be an iterative process that includes various stakeholder perspectives (students, staff, families) as well as routine data analysis.
- Schools should carefully select prevention and intervention approaches to match the needs of their student populations. In turn, scholarly research should assess the effectiveness of promotion, prevention and intervention efforts across contexts, in order to build an evidence base of culturally validated intervention strategies

Reflection points and questions

This section promotes the discussion of ideas that can lead to a *shared agenda* (Andis et al. 2002), in which leaders, staff and stakeholders from education, mental health, other youth serving systems, and families and youth meet to develop relationships and build support for school mental health across dimensions of training, practice, research and policy (Weist and Murray 2007). The following list of questions can help promote school–community dialogue about strengthening school mental health through a public health framework.

- What are some of the key advantages of instituting a public mental health model within schools? Reflect on how a public health approach to school mental health can address some of the issues schools currently experience (i.e. need to raise achievement, issues with bullying, insufficient resources to address needs of all students, etc.).
- What are specific ways that school mental health providers can collaborate with educators to implement a full continuum of promotion, prevention and intervention efforts within the school?
- How can students, families, teachers and community stakeholders be engaged to provide input on needs and strengths and recommendations to establish and continuously improve school mental health?

Further reading and resources

Table 14.1 contains links to a wide range of international resources. In addition, an example of a well-used online mental health curriculum can be found at www.mindreel.org.uk.

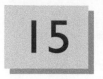

15 Mental health and wellbeing at the workplace

Eva Jané-Llopis and Cary L Cooper

Burden and costs of mental ill health in the workplace: the imperative for action

Lack of wellbeing and mental ill health: an intangible burden

Employment is generally beneficial to physical and mental health, the main source of income for most people and a defining feature of social status (McDaid 2008). Structuring employment to create 'good work' brings health benefits to the individual, financial benefits to the corporation and both direct and indirect improvements to the fabric of society.

Although in some cases the working environment can have an adverse impact on mental health, there is general acceptance that the nature of work and the way that it is organized dictates whether it is likely to benefit or to harm the health and wellbeing of workers (Lundberg and Cooper 2011).

The current severe economic downturn has had a terrible impact on wellbeing, and has disproportionately affected workers at either end of the age spectrum as well as those with disability (Stuckler et al. 2011). Strong evidence also indicates that the risk of unemployment and loss of employment are associated with an increased rate of harmful stress, anxiety, depression and psychotic disorders (WHO 2010). The global financial situation and the increased instability in employment has also had an indirect impact on how stress and lack of wellbeing are experienced.

Occupational stress and work-related mental health problems have a number of major socio-economic consequences such as absenteeism, labour turnover, loss of productivity and disability pension costs (Palmer and Dryden 1994; Dewe and Kompier 2008). Personal costs include lower self-esteem, physical conditions (for example heart disease) and a negative impact on family life (Goodspeed and DeLucia 1990). For these reasons, the workplace is considered to be one of the most important settings for mental health promotion.

Mental disorders are the most important cause of disability in all regions of the world, accounting for around one-third of years lived with disability among adults aged 15 years and over (WHO 2008). Furthermore, unlike most chronic illnesses, the age distribution is relatively constant with adults of working age being as likely to suffer as those who are older. Overall, one in four people in employment can expect to experience some kind of mental health problem once during their lifetime.

Costs of mental ill health

Impaired mental health accounts for tremendous costs to society and businesses. The economic cost to society is substantial: depression alone is estimated as absorbing 1 per cent of Europe's gross domestic product (Sobocki et al. 2006); globally, mental ill health is estimated to account for a cumulative US$16 trillion of global output loss in the next 20 years (Bloom et al. 2011). For individual companies mental health is now often the commonest cause of sickness absence in richer countries, accounting for 30 to 50 per cent of all new disability benefit claims in OECD countries (OECD 2011b), for up to 40 per cent of time lost (Cooper and Dewe 2008) and with presenteeism (lost productivity while at work) adding at least 1.5 times to the cost of absenteeism (Parsonage 2007). Similarly, other non-communicable diseases, especially, cardiovascular disease, cancer, diabetes and respiratory diseases follow suit with an estimated cumulative output loss in the next 20 years of over US$30 trillion (Bloom et al. 2011) due to direct and indirect costs to employers and society as a whole.

Work-related stress and poor mental health are major reasons not only for absenteeism but also for occupational disability and for workers seeking early retirement (WHO 2010). This is a growing financial strain across countries, as young people in many countries increasingly enter the disability benefit system without having spent much time in the workforce, meaning the population claiming disability benefits is getting younger in most countries (OECD 2011b). See Box 15.1 for estimated costs in England.

Box 15.1 Economic and social costs of mental ill health

Taking England as an example, it has been estimated that the economic and social costs of mental ill health were over £105 billion in 2009, of which some £30 billion relate to the costs of output losses resulting from the adverse effects of mental health problems on people's ability to work (Centre for Mental Health 2011). Along these lines, the annual cost of mental ill health to employers in the UK is significant, estimated at £25.9 billion in 2006 or £28.3 billion at 2009 pay levels (Foresight Mental Capital and Well-being project – Dewe and Kompier 2008; NICE 2009c). The £25.9 billion can be broken down as £8.4 billion a year for sickness absence, £15.1 billion a year for reduced productivity at work and £2.4 billion a year for turnover, replacing staff who leave their jobs because of mental ill health.

During economic recession and the implementation of austerity measures, public and private sector spending are carefully considered and cuts are made in areas not considered a priority. Preventive action and mental health services often suffer and their capacity may paradoxically be reduced at times of increased need (WHO 2010).

Causes for psychosocial stress at the workplace

As reiterated by the WHO (2010), individual reactions to the same psychosocial exposure may vary. For example, high commitment and a high need for approval influence people's perceptions of job demand and their own coping resources (Wilkinson and Marmot 2003; Marmot and

Wilkinson 2006). Some people can cope with high demands and high levels of psychosocial risk factors; others cannot. The subjective evaluation of the situation is always decisive for the stress reaction. However, several factors that are common across individuals have been established as known sources and causes of stress and stress-related illness at work (WHO 2010, Box 15.2) that can be efficiently targeted by evidence-based interventions.

> **Box 15.2 Some key factors that lead to stress at work**
> **(adapted from WHO 2010)**
>
> • High demands and low control.
> • Lack of control and poor decision-making latitude.
> • Low social support.
> • Imbalance between effort and reward.
> • Monotony.
> • Poor communication and information.
> • Unclear or ambiguous instructions and role, unclear organizational and personal goals.
> • Lack of participation.
> • Emotionally distressing human services work such as healthcare or teaching.
> • Job insecurity.
> • Time pressure.
> • Bullying, harassment and violence.
> • Organizational change.

Effective action in promoting workplace mental health and wellbeing

Many of the new generation of workplace wellness initiatives are made up of a complementary package of interventions aiming to prevent non-communicable diseases including stress and mental ill health. These programmes address a common set of underlying modifiable behavioural risk factors that can prevent as much as 80 per cent of cardiovascular disease and 40 per cent of cancers (Gaziano et al. 2010). Both the underlying risk factors (tobacco and harmful use of alcohol, poor diet and lack of physical activity) as well as the non-communicable diseases they cause, are highly comorbid with mental disorders and are responsible for additive increase in work-loss (Buist-Bouwman et al. 2005). Workplace programmes that address these risk factors have proven effective and cost-effective in reducing risks and the overall burden of non-communicable diseases and related mental health problems. Programmes report different levels of efficacy (Baicker et al. 2010).

Likewise, evidence from recent systematic reviews indicates that effective actions for preventing stress and mental ill health in the workplace can be implemented successfully both at an organizational level within the workplace and targeted at specific individuals (Dewe and Kompier 2008; McDaid 2008; WHO 2010; Czabala et al. 2011). However, such results are maintained only when we ensure sustainable implementation of those programmes proven effective; we support adherence to the programme; and we provide incentives for follow-up measures (WHO and World Economic Forum 2008).

Organizational-level actions and management of work

Programmes with the largest impact are those that target an organizational change through the promotion of awareness among managers of the importance of mental health and wellbeing at work; the improvement of their skills in risk management for stress and poor mental health; and the creation of supportive work content, environments and management styles. Effective work content protects employees from unreasonable job demands, and promotes employee control and autonomy, flexible working schedules and job stability. Effective management styles promote organizational justice, workplace support, active participation of employees and provide clear and consistent communication.

The management of work

The way that people are managed at work has a profound influence on their wellbeing. It is a compelling indictment of some modern management practice, that in many countries there is an increase in management-related bullying in the workplace (Einarsen et al. 2011). Although studies suggest that the time workers enjoy least in the day is time spent with their line manager (Kahnemnan 2004), conversely, a consistent finding of employee engagement surveys highlights that the line manager is the most trusted source of information in the workplace. Some companies are seeking to redress this shortcoming, and a set of management competencies has been developed by the UK's Health and Safety Executive (HSE), in conjunction with the Chartered Institute of Personnel and Development and Investors in People (HSE 2009), to define the behaviours identified as effective for preventing and reducing stress at work (see Table 15.1).

Table 15.1 Effective behaviours to prevent and reduce stress at work

Competency	Subcompetency
Respectful and responsible: managing emotions and having integrity	Integrity *Being respectful and honest to employees* Managing emotions *Behaving consistently and calmly around the team* Considerate approach *Being thoughtful in managing others and delegating*
Managing and communicating existing and future work	Proactive work management *Monitoring and reviewing existing work, allowing future prioritization and planning* Problem-solving *Dealing with problems promptly, rationally and responsibly* Participative/empowering *Listening to, meeting and consulting with the team, providing direction, autonomy and development opportunities to individuals*
Managing the individual within the team	Personally accessible *Available to talk to personally* Sociable *Relaxed approach, such as socializing and using humour* Empathetic engagement *Seeking to understand each individual in the team in terms of their health and satisfaction, motivation, point of view and life outside work*
Reasoning/managing difficult situations	Managing conflict *Dealing with conflicts decisively, promptly and objectively* Use of organizational resources *Seeking advice when necessary from managers, human resources and occupational health* Taking responsibility for resolving issues *Having a supportive and responsible approach to issues and incidents in the team*

Individual-level programmes

For individuals, effective comprehensive programmes are those that promote both resilience and stress management (Robertson and Cooper 2011). These programmes targeting individual approaches vary greatly and can include: modifying workloads, providing CBT, relaxation and meditation training, time management training, exercise programmes, journaling, biofeedback and goal setting (Czabala et al. 2011). Enhancing the wellbeing of employees and providing information about mental health issues has a beneficial impact on families and communities as well as enhancing the organization in terms of increased productivity and turnover. For example, it has been estimated that effective management of mental health in a UK organization with 100 employees could save £250,000 per year (NICE 2009c).

Combined programmes – stress awareness and management programmes

Multi-component awareness and stress management programmes that combine interventions to help individuals deal with work-related stress and organizational measures to deal with risk factors and structural issues of content and quality of work are highly effective preventive measures and benefit business productivity (Semmer 2008). These approaches are particularly recommended given the high success rate of individual approaches and the lack of sustained effects of some organizational-level only measures, which at times depend on external factors (Semmer 2008). To support this, a strong role in these programmes can be played by managerial staff, such as line managers and workers' representatives, whose skills and awareness of work-related stress and mental health issues can be strengthened while working on developing an environment where people feel empowered and comfortable talking about mental health issues. Programmes might also involve the use of specialist trainers or facilitators whose aim is to enhance the resilience and coping skills of individuals in dealing with stressful situations, managing their time or deal with harassment in the workplace (McDaid 2011).

Return on investment

Although it has been proven that workplace initiatives can yield significant benefits, the science on return on investment (ROI) is still young and because different methodologies are used to ascertain cost–benefits of interventions, making comparisons remains difficult. Some studies attempting to calculate the ROI suffer from either lack of a control group or a bias with regard to participants, size of employers or a strong focus on positive results (World Economic Forum 2012). However, although generally evidence points to medium to large returns for workplace health promotion overall, including programmes targeting mental health, estimates from specific ROI studies vary as widely as a return of US$165 to US$970 on every dollar spent (World Economic Forum 2012).

For example, a recent review produced by the UK Department of Health modelled the costs of a multi-component health promotion intervention composed of: personalized health and wellbeing information and advice; a health risk appraisal questionnaire; access to a tailored health improvement web portal; wellness literature; and seminars and workshops focused on identified wellness issues (Knapp et al. 2011). The cost of such multi-component intervention was estimated at £80 per employee per year, and, modelling costs/savings in a white collar enterprise with 500 employees, and taking into account uptake of the intervention (43 per cent of all employees) and impact on absenteeism and presenteeism, in year 1, the initial costs of £40,000 for the programme were outweighed by gains arising from reduced presenteeism and absenteeism of £387,722. This represents a substantial annual return on investment of more than nine to one (Knapp et al. 2011).

Using another economic modulation developed by Healthways and the Boston Consulting Group, it was estimated that US companies could save an average of US$700 per year and employee on healthcare costs and productivity gained if they were to address inactivity, stress and harmful use of alcohol over five years (World Economic Forum 2010a). Although these savings in healthcare costs are specific to the USA, increase in productivity can be achieved across countries. For example, in a model calculation for 10,000 employees, a cost of intervention of US$8 per employee per month would yield an overall ROI potential of 390–755 per cent, depending on location (World Economic Forum 2010a).

A recent Harvard-led meta-analysis, which reviewed 36 studies for analytical rigour, identifies an average ROI of US$3.27 for every dollar spent on wellness programmes (Baicker et al. 2010). Robust reviews suggest that although ROI may vary due to different factors ranging from how the programme is set up to the broader cultural and regional context, there is a measurable return for many of the dollars spent globally on these programmes.

From practice to evidence: addressing the new challenges in workplace mental health and wellbeing

The current evidence base on the value of workplace wellness raises several questions: how best should a programme be evaluated? What concrete return will a particular programme deliver? What are the real costs of lost productivity and how best can we measure it? How does the health and wellbeing of my organization compare with similar organizations? How can success be monitored and encouraged? Some of the new challenges in workplace mental health and wellbeing will require a joint effort that brings together the private sector and academia in strong partnerships, and ultimately the public sector in their role as employers.

For example, although workplace wellness programmes seem to be effective, there appears to be a mismatch between what is being undertaken by many businesses, particularly the larger multinationals, and the clear lack of published evaluations in this space. This leads to a vacuum in the evidence base or a lag in insight about these practices, because more is being done than is actually published or shared. Integral to the development of workplace programmes is the need for embedded evaluation and tracking metrics of the impact of those programmes, as some organizations have started doing (Table 15.1 and Box 15.3). Partnerships between workplaces and academia to support strong evaluations and reporting on the outcomes would provide a richness of data urgently needed to strengthen the business case.

Box 15.3 Case study from British Telecom: a measured approach to better mental health

Tracking metrics is an integral part of the way that the company manages its business and mental health is no exception. The company's 'Positive Mentality' mental health promotion programme had evaluation built in from the start. A total of 51 per cent of people who participated reported an improvement in their mental wellbeing and 34 per cent reported they had learned something new about mental health. The mental wellbeing of the workforce is monitored continuously and reported monthly to senior management through a mental health dashboard. The dashboard takes feeds from the sickness absence, occupational health, employee assistance and stress assessment databases to give a picture, down to divisional level, of the extent, severity and work causes for impaired mental health. Management, supported by the company psychologist, use the information to develop and refine tailored mental health action plans for each part of the business. This approach has helped to mitigate the impact on employees of very difficult economic circumstances.

There is, in addition, a need for sharing of metrics and progress in real work environments to gain further intelligence on the efficiency and pay-offs of these practices and how they benchmark against each other. A recent initiative has started an attempt to standardize, collect and share employee metrics at a global level, and although many difficulties lay ahead, it is critical that future partnerships develop in this area (World Economic Forum 2011).

Likewise, the efficiency of programmes could be maximized. Many workplaces are targeting the prevention of non-communicable diseases, and, given the similarity of programme components and large comorbidities, there is enormous opportunity to integrate actions that tackle physical health, and particularly non-communicable diseases, with promoting mental health and wellbeing at work, as many of the competences apply to both and are mutually beneficial.

Whereas the costs of dealing with poor mental health have been the focus of attention by policy makers in recent years (Dewa et al. 2007), less attention has been given to evaluating the economic costs and benefits of promoting positive mental health in the workplace. In part, this may be due to a lack of incentives for business to undertake such evaluations, or due to issues of commercial sensitivity. Looking into ROI is critical and such studies are urgently needed. Alongside reporting on cost–benefits of interventions, evaluations should also calculate the objective loss that lack of productivity brings. This might be already done at the corporate level and not reported, but further studies and evidence are urgently needed to strengthen the evidence base as well as the business case for workplace wellness. For example, a recent study in a company setting within a real work environment has shown how workgroups with higher levels of depressive symptoms had significantly poorer work performance and how computer-aided web-based screening for symptoms of depression is feasible in a work setting (Harvey et al. 2011).

The opportunity lies ahead

Providing a healthy and inclusive working environment can prevent mental health problems and enhance opportunities to enter, remain at or return to work when experiencing such problems. Good health contributes to quality and productivity at work, which in turn promotes economic growth and employment (McDaid 2011) and the ability to invest in good employment practices.

Organizations can avoid considerable costs by managing their operations in a way that promotes wellbeing among their workers. However, that is only part of the prize to be gained because happy and healthy employees are more innovative, more productive and relate better to customers (World Economic Forum 2010b). Engagement without wellbeing leads to a burned-out workforce where talent retention is poor (Robertson and Cooper 2011). The strong case of improving wellbeing in the workplace can be made not only to businesses but to the public sector, including the NHS as well, as it has been shown that the benefits as an employer from improved investment in workplace wellbeing programmes applies to private and public sectors alike (Knapp et al. 2011). And, in spite of the ROI, the outset of such programmes does not require large expenses. Spreitzer and Porath (2012) specify that thriving employees consistently show up at work, make major contributions and are in it for the long haul; and they state that encouraging all employees to thrive requires concerted attention, not huge financial resources. This phenomenon is increasingly recognized by investors seeking long-term returns, and analysts have largely driven the movement to encourage publicly listed companies to report on employee wellbeing (Anderson et al. 2011).

In addressing these new challenges posed by the new nature of jobs and societal changes, new opportunities will have to be sought and evaluated thoroughly. For example, rapid advances in information and communication technology have ended the requirement for many workers to be tied to a specific location and they can now often fulfil their roles effectively from an alternative workplace, home or while on the move. The resulting benefits to wellbeing for the worker, not least as a result of reduced commuting, are matched by opportunities for the employer to improve efficiency and to rationalize property requirements and have yielded substantial benefit-to-cost ratios for organizations (Cooper et al. 2010). Our current and new ways of working and understanding of wellbeing open up new directions and interesting challenges for the field of workplace health that will only be addressed if stronger partnerships and collaborations are developed.

As long ago as 1968 Robert Kennedy gave a speech at the University of Kansas contrasting the contributions of gross national product (GNP) and wellbeing to the national debate, which has relevance to the happiness/wellbeing at work agenda seen in many countries:

Too much and for too long, we seemed to have surrendered personal excellence and community values in the mere accumulation of material things. Our Gross National Product, now, is over $800b a year, but that GNP—if we judge the USA by that—that GNP counts air pollution and cigarette advertising, and the ambulances to clear our highways of carnage. It counts special locks for our doors and the jails for the people who break them. It counts the destruction of the redwood and the loss of our natural wonder in chaotic sprawl. It counts napalm and counts warheads and armoured cars for the police to fight the riots in our cities ... Yet the GNP does not allow for the health of our children, the quality of their education or the job of their play. It does not include the beauty of our poetry or the strength of our marriages, the intelligence of our public debate or the integrity of our public officials. It measures neither our wit nor our courage, neither our wisdom nor our learning, neither our compassion nor our devotion to our country. It measures everything in short, except that which makes life worthwhile.
(Kennedy, 1968: para. 23)

Mini toolkit

Top tips for effective practice

- Decide what the focus of your programme is – promotion of wellbeing for all staff, prevention of stress or mental distress, or support for those with mental illness – and ensure there are appropriate interventions and evaluation measures in the planning stages.
- All initiatives should be developed in partnership with employees and their representative organizations.
- Programmes should be sustainable and mainstreamed into workplace policies if they are effective.

Case study

See Box 15.3 for a case study from British Telecom.

Undertaking research and evaluation

More advanced health impact assessments are required to evaluate the wider benefits of workplace mental health programmes at the individual, organizational and social levels. This requires strong partnerships between universities and public, private and NGOs. Research should focus upon:

- the wellbeing of all employees including the recruitment and retention of people with mental health problems;
- the concrete returns that programmes deliver to employers;
- how workplace mental health initiatives affect the wider community.

Reflection points and questions

- To what extent can we leave businesses to lead efforts to improve employee health and reduce disparities?
- When is work bad for mental health?
- To what extent might a workplace's aims to promote positive mental health for all of its employees be more effective in supporting people with severe mental health problems to gain and sustain employment?

Further reading and resources

- Organisation for Economic Co-operation and Development: Better Life Initiative: Measuring Well-being and Progress, available at www.oecd.org/statistics/betterlife-initiativemeasuringwell-beingandprogress.htm (accessed 28 August 2012).
- UK Government Foresight Report 'Mental Capital and Wellbeing' available at http://www.bis.gov.uk/foresight/our-work/projects/published-projects/mental-capital-and-wellbeing/reports-and-publications (accessed 28 August 2012).
- World Economic Forum Wellness Initiatives: www.weforum.org/issues/workplace-wellness-alliance (accessed 28 August 2012).
- European Network for Workplace Health Promotion: Work in tune with life, available at www.oefi.hu/lelekrehangolva/employer.pdf (accessed 28 August 2012) has tools for detailed planning of interventions.

Acknowledgements

The authors greatly acknowledge the support, input and resources of Dr Paul Litchfield, Chief Medical Officer at British Telecom.

16 Later life

Mima Cattan

Introduction

We are living in an ageing world. The demographic changes facing most countries resulting from lower birth rates and increased longevity means that older people and old age cannot be ignored. By 2030, about 25 per cent of the population in many European countries will be aged 65 years and over. The greatest increase will occur in the number and proportion of people aged 80+. The number of 'very old' people is projected to double in the UK from 4.5 per cent in 2008 to 9 per cent in 2060 but almost triple in several other European countries in the same time period (Giannakouris 2008; Office for National Statistics 2011). This will have major implications for public health policy, resources and services.

Old age defined

There is no general agreement on 'old age'. The UN has a cut-off of 60+ years to refer to older people, but many countries have selected an arbitrary chronological age of 60 or 65 years as the age when people retire (WHO 2011a). However, in many developing countries changes in social role and function are far more relevant 'markers' into old age than a retirement age, and such changes may come about much earlier than at 60 or 65. Chronological ageing as a social construct therefore has different meanings in different countries, societies and cultures. Viewed as a social construct, chronological age may be more attuned to a person's functional age, i.e. the functional decline that occurs over the lifespan, rather than simply the number of years the person has lived.

Chronological age is particularly misleading when it comes to mental health. Although some mental health problems, such as dementia, seem to increase with age, this does not mean that they are inevitable consequences of ageing. Consequently, the concept of old age is a fusion of chronological, functional and social factors, with the building blocks for mental health in later life including physical health, the availability of social support and social networks, security and 'happiness'.

The importance of life-course

Older people are probably a more diverse group than any other age group, simply because they have lived longer and have accumulated experiences through the life-course. A person's life-course can be viewed as the social element of their lifespan, marked by a number of life transitions, some being clear 'stages' through life, and others significant planned or unplanned life events (Hubley and Copeman 2008; Hutchinson 2011). Older people can differ in age from 60 years upwards, belong to different ethnic and religious groups, and have varying levels of education, income and affluence and health. Their experiences, personal and living circumstances, sexuality, culture and values can be different. Their roles in society are diverse: they may be grandparents, in employment, in prison, caregivers or homeless. Placed in an ecological and societal framework all these factors are relevant in a public health context and pose challenges in the promotion of mental health.

Mental health and wellbeing in later life

As seen in previous chapters, there is a myriad of definitions relating to public mental health and wellbeing. The WHO's definition: 'a state of well-being in which every individual realizes his or her own potential, can cope with the normal stresses of life, can work productively and fruitfully, and is able to make a contribution to her or his community' (WHO 2011b: para. 2) excludes many older people. They may be perfectly mentally healthy without necessarily contributing directly to their community or working productively. If we accept that good mental health is a right of all older people, we can consider public mental health from two perspectives: older people's views on mental health and the determinants of mental health.

Research has shown that older people define mental health and wellbeing as personal resources (for example good health, ability to adjust, freedom from stress and worries), individual characteristics (for example self-esteem, self-efficacy, independence and control), environmental resources (for example availability of support from social networks, safe environment), and attitudes (to keep involved with change, to keep busy) (Giuntoli and Cattan 2010). When asked what promotes mental health, they mention environmental resources, people's attitudes and individual characteristics. They emphasize the importance of reciprocity and having a role in life, being able to maintain confidence and to cope with loss, and the impact of ageism.

The determinants of mental health and older people

The determinants of health have been grouped into socioeconomic factors, environment, health behaviours, and biological and personal factors (European Union Public Health Information and Knowledge System (EUPHIX) 2009). Based on research with older people, this framework can also be used to describe the wider determinants of mental health in later life, highlighting the main issues that public mental health needs to consider: retirement and financial security; physical, sensory and cognitive decline and ways of maintaining active ageing; social connectedness and social exclusion; the built and green environment. Each of these areas will now be discussed.

Retirement and financial security

The issues

A man retiring in the UK at the age of 60 can now expect 18.1 years of retirement, whereas a woman retiring at the same age can expect up to 22.1 years (ONS 2011b). This will have long-term implications for retirement pensions, health and social care. Several governments have moved towards raising the state pension age. In the UK, the state pension age will rise in stages to 67 by 2028, and the Government has proposed that in the future, the state pension age should be based on demographic evidence of life expectancy. Particularly for women on low incomes this could mean added hardship as they get older, and a retirement of financial insecurity. We know that income security is influenced by several inter-related factors, for example gender, social class, occupation, ethnicity and health status (Moffatt 2009), that have an impact on mental wellbeing.

Retirement is one of several key transition points over the life-course, which can have an impact on people's health. Cumulative disadvantage through the life-course is more likely to lead to poverty, social exclusion and physical and mental ill health (McKee et al. 2010), resulting in widening inequalities with age. Chandola et al. (2007) found that although mental health generally improved with age in all occupational groups, those in higher occupational groups attained better mental health after retirement. The relationship between retirement, socio-economic status and mental health is, however, not linear. It seems that having control over one's working conditions *before* retirement and being able to decide when and how to leave work are major factors in determining a person's mental health in retirement (Leinonen et al. 2011). It is likely that individuals who perceive being in control over their financial situation, have high occupational status and good social support have better resources for mental health (Wilkinson and Marmot 2003) than those forced to retire early on health grounds or through redundancy.

The solutions

With such deep-rooted problems, it might seem almost impossible to find effective solutions to improve older people's mental health through financial interventions, other than to increase the amount of money paid in pensions. This may indeed be the main solution in developing countries. A universal social pension for all older people is seen by many as a basic human right, to reduce poverty and achieve greater equity (HelpAge International 2006).

In countries, with state pensions, there is still inequity in accessing additional benefits for pensioners living in poverty. In the UK a large proportion of benefits are not claimed because of lack of knowledge and the complexity of the system and other barriers. The lack of uptake can be tackled through information campaigns to alert older people to the existence of benefits, and the provision of individually tailored benefits advice. Such interventions can help to increase older people's uptake of benefits and improve their wellbeing (Moffatt and Scambler 2008). Supplementary finances can help older people to deal with day-to-day outgoings, and cope with one-off emergencies, making their lives more manageable, increasing their independence and quality of life. Many local Age UK organizations now have volunteers providing benefits advice for older people in their own homes.

Physical, sensory and cognitive decline – maintaining active ageing

The issues

Research suggests that physical activity has a positive impact on mental wellbeing and cognitive function. Generally, physical activity levels drop with age. However, those who have been active during their working life are more likely to continue being active in their old age (Soule et al. 2005). Although the processes involved in improving mental health through physical activity are not fully understood, physical activity is associated with improvements in physical health (Clow and Aitchison 2009), which in turn can affect mental wellbeing.

Sensory impairment is more common in older people. There is increasing evidence that both vision and hearing impairments have a greater impact on health outcomes than was previously thought (Capella-McDonnall 2005; Hogan et al. 2009). Mobility is of particular concern to older people with sight loss, frequently resulting in withdrawal from social activities, and increased social isolation and loneliness (Cattan et al. 2010). The links between sight loss and depression are well documented (Fletcher et al. 2008). Older people with sensory loss face the same life transitions through loss and decline in health as those who are sighted, but in addition, they have to cope with the special challenges of sight and hearing loss. For many this means no longer being able to engage in activities they have previously found meaningful and enjoyed.

The solutions

'Active ageing' is promoted as one of the main policies for maintaining mental wellbeing (Lang et al. 2010; WHO 2011c). The WHO's definition of active ageing emphasizes the ability to participate in society, healthy life expectancy and quality of life. Unsurprisingly, the evidence base for such a broad theme is rather mixed. Most research to date has focused on the impact of physical activity on older people's mental health (Windle et al. 2010), with NICE recommending community-based tailored physical activity programmes, walking groups and training for active daily living to promote older people's mental wellbeing (NICE 2008b). However, the diversity of old age and the pre-requisites for older people to be able to participate in such activities is rarely taken into account.

Social connectedness and social exclusion

The issues

Social connectedness refers to the connections and relationships people have with others in their environment. Older people experience social exclusion when they lack access to social networks, services and activities leading to a poor quality of life (Social Exclusion Unit 2006). Exclusion is also linked to economic and material deprivation, low educational attainment and mental health problems. For older people the cumulative effect of adverse life events and age discrimination can compound the impact of social exclusion, resulting in depression and other mental health problems. Depression is directly associated with social isolation and loneliness.

Although loneliness can be experienced at any age, older people are at greater risk of enduring loneliness, because of a reduction in personal and external resources available to them. Loneliness has been described as a mismatch between one's desired level of companionship and the relationships one has. Loneliness is associated with a wide range of physical and mental health problems and with a reduction in quality of life (Bowling and Gabriel 2007). Loneliness can occur as a result of one event, such as the loss of one's partner, or it can be chronic and made worse by transitions into old age. Research shows that between 30 and 40 per cent of older people in the UK and other European countries are sometimes or often lonely (Victor et al. 2009), and this figure has remained fairly constant for the past 40 years. With the increase in the numbers of people aged 60+, the actual numbers of older people experiencing loneliness are also increasing. Known risk factors include loss and bereavement, widowhood, perceived and actual poor health, lack of resources, living alone and time spent alone (Scharf and De Jong Gierveld 2008). The risk of suicide increases in older people who are lonely and depressed (Koponen et al. 2007).

The solutions

It has been proposed that some basic 'rights' need to be in place to reduce social exclusion among older people: acceptable standards of health and wealth, access to social activities and support, adequate housing, access to transport and reduced age discrimination and fear of crime (Social Exclusion Unit 2006). Some of these suggestions require government policy action, whereas others can be initiated locally.

Volunteering has been put forward as a way of improving older people's mental health and reducing social exclusion (von Bonsdorff and Rantanen 2010). The number of older volunteers is increasing in many European countries, because of better health, increased life expectancy and more leisure time. Older people volunteer to meet new people, to do something meaningful and help others and to 'give something back' (GHK 2010). Although volunteering may help to improve *some* older people's quality of life, little is known about who actually benefits, the social and cultural context of volunteering and its role in reducing inequalities (Cattan et al. 2011a).

A systematic review of interventions alleviating loneliness showed that effective interventions shared several characteristics: they were group activities with an educational input of some type or provided specific support activities; they were established for specific groups; they enabled some participant control or consulted with the intended target group; they were established within an existing service (Cattan et al. 2005). Befriending schemes, face to face or telephone, have received increased attention. Research suggests that lonely older people value having someone to talk to about everyday things. A regular telephone call can be a lifeline for housebound older people and help them to gain confidence, re-engage with the community and become socially active again (Cattan et al. 2011b). The value of other technologies for older people, such as email, the internet and social networking sites are yet to be evaluated.

The environment, housing and transport

The issues

There is a body of research linking mental health with the environment. Poor housing can contribute to raised stress and depression (Lang et al. 2010), busy roads, lack of appropriate public transport or fear of being injured as a result of bus driver carelessness can result in social isolation (Marsden et al. 2010), and the availability of urban green space can have an impact on mental health. Although the association between housing, transport and mental health is fairly clear, less is known about the interaction between green space and mental wellbeing. Theoretical models for health promoting pathways linking environment and health are underdeveloped and there is a lack of consensus about what measures of effect should be considered (Pinder et al. 2009).

The solutions

Most proposed solutions to improve mental health through environmental change are based on limited knowledge about the associations between mental health and the environment. An EU conference on older people's mental health (Lang et al. 2010) stressed that the provision of a wide range of housing options with a strong infrastructure is essential for older people's quality of life. Access to reliable and safe public transport, well-lit pavements, crime-free environments and spaces for people to walk and interact with others is also said to be important for older people's wellbeing (Gilhooly 2002; Day 2008; Schipperijn et al. 2010), but such interventions are yet to be evaluated.

Conclusions

This chapter has considered the main public mental health issues for older people through a life-course perspective. Until recently, the promotion of older people's mental health mainly focused on the prevention of ill health in individuals rather than on the wider determinants of public health, resulting in older people's mental wellbeing frequently being neglected or completely ignored. As people age, they continue to interact with others and with the environment around them. Public mental health promotion has the capacity to recognize that not only do older people have a human right to wellbeing, but that their health also has an impact on the wellbeing of others around them.

As this chapter has demonstrated, the evidence for wider public mental health interventions is still limited, and tends to focus on individual or single activity interventions. Older people have often been excluded from research on wider public health issues, such as transport or housing. Through increased understanding of the factors that have an impact on older people's mental health, we should in the future be able to design and evaluate complex public health interventions across the life-course that include older people.

Mini toolkit

Top tips for effective practice

Consider the following points when developing public mental health programmes for older people:

- inclusivity – the benefits of using a life-course approach;
- specific issues related to ageing;
- involvement – draw on older people's experiences and perspectives in the development and implementation of meaningful programmes.

Case study

The provision of advice and support on how to access and claim benefits can be a simple and low-cost public health intervention, which improves older people's quality of life, by helping them to manage their day-to-day lives. The strength of the intervention is that it can be provided in any service accessed by older people and adapted to their personal needs. It draws on the principles of human rights and Amartya Sen's (1988) argument that income inequality is not just about what people have (such as the right to benefits) but also what they are able to do with what they have (can they access the benefits and how can the benefits be put to best use for them).

Undertaking research and evaluation

Public mental health and older people is an under-researched area. Research in this field will increasingly require complex interdisciplinary intervention studies and studies that investigate the interactions between factors known to have an impact on mental health. Local evaluations should:

- involve older people in the entire evaluation process;
- be clear about their definitions of 'mental health' and 'older people';
- be prepared to use a variety of methods that will answer the questions being posed and are realistic within available resources and time frame.

Reflection points and questions

- Consider the advantages and disadvantages of using chronological age when addressing older people's mental health.
- Reflect on why older people are often discriminated against in mental health promotion, and how this could be redressed.
- On the basis of current evidence, what might the most far-reaching interventions for maintaining older people's mental health be.
- Reflect on how 'active ageing' could be used to promote older people's mental health.
- Accepting that most older people will have some decline in their physical health, consider what this might mean for a population and/or a life-course approach in public mental health promotion.

Further reading and resources

- Age Concern (2006) *Promoting Mental Health and Well-being in Later Life*. London: Mental Health Foundation.
- Campaign to End Loneliness (2011) See: http://www.campaigntoendloneliness.org.uk/ (accessed 28 August 2012).
- Cattan, M. (ed) (2009) *Mental Health and Well-being in Later Life*. Maidenhead: McGraw-Hill/Open University Press.
- Cattan, M. (2010) *Preventing Social Isolation and Loneliness among Older People*. Saarbrucken: Lambert Academic Publishing.
- Hubley, J. and Copeman, J. (2008) *Practical Health Promotion,* at www.polity.co.uk/health-promotion/ (accessed 28 August 2012).
- Johnson, M.L. (ed) (2005) *The Cambridge Handbook of Age and Ageing*. Cambridge: Cambridge University Press.
- Vincent, J., Phillipson, C. and Downs, M. (eds) (2006) *The Futures of Old Age*. London: Sage.

MONKLANDS HOSPITAL
LIBRARY
MONKSCOURT AVENUE
AIRDRIE ML60JS
☎ 01236712005

17 Lessons and directions for public mental health

Neil Quinn and Lee Knifton

Chapter contents

Equity	Communities of practice
Determinants	International action
Empowering individuals and communities	

What emerges throughout this book is that improving the public's mental health is a dynamic and complex area. To present it as a simple narrative would not do justice to the scale of the challenge or the range and quality of the work that has been developed. By taking a broad view of public mental health, we have introduced a rich analysis of the key issues. Our authors are leaders in their respective fields and are drawn from across different disciplines, demonstrating at a very fundamental level that the challenges of public mental health can only be fully understood and addressed by a multidisciplinary approach.

The book is not only multidisciplinary but introduces ideas and approaches from authors adopting different theoretical standpoints. One dimension that recurs throughout the chapters is the relationship between the individual–society or agency–structure. Many authors stress the significance of social context in determining public mental health, and they focus upon changing social structures, institutions, economic resources and cultures. This is exemplified in the chapter by Mathieson and colleagues, which looks at regeneration and community building. Others stress the importance of individual action or agency, for example Maxwell on preventing depression and Reavley and Jorm's mental health literacy work, where emphasis is placed upon the cumulative actions of individuals having an impact on interpersonal and wider community life. These positions, in turn, shape the way in which we gather our evidence and develop our evaluations. We can see this if we contrast Stewart-Brown's focus upon the individual and Pickett and Wilkinson's focus upon structural measures. We believe that although it is important to acknowledge the theoretical (and often highly political) underpinnings of your approach, we must be pragmatic. Individuals and society are interconnected and can only be understood in relation to one another. Public mental health programmes and evaluations must operate at multiple levels – from individual and group through to community, organizations and wider society. This pragmatic position is adopted by most of our authors.

Several chapters highlight the limits of biomedicine and positivistic positions in public mental health. Theorists often talk of the art, science and politics of public health (see Friedli 2004) but at a basic level this really echoes the recurrent debates across social sciences. Without rehearsing these arguments, and again explicitly stating that our position is a pragmatic one, it is sufficient to highlight that public mental health practice and research should take account of, if not be embedded in, post-positivist and social constructionist theories. The de-/reconstructing of mental illness categories, the conceptualization of mental health and illness as a single or dual continuum, the concept of recovery as a parallel or master narrative over psychiatry (as articulated so well by Mary O'Hagan), and the sociocultural meanings people attach to mental illness within and between communities – have all been central to the evolution of our discipline.

What is important though is that the book offers a wide range of differing perspectives but still manages to offer clear directions for taking forward the public mental health agenda – a point that is reinforced by the toolkits and practical resources sections. But compared with many other areas of public health identifying achievements remains challenging. This is partly due to the fact that this is an emerging area, but also the fact that it can be very complex to capture impact with complete confidence. Many interventions are recent and research and evaluation tools are underdeveloped compared with other areas of public health. Moreover, there can be a multiplicity of factors that influence mental health outcomes. So although many areas now have valuable evidence to justify and inform programmes, this is still emerging. This is illustrated in the chapters on suicide prevention by Beautrais and Larkin or stigma reduction by Rüsch and Corrigan, where the complexities of evaluating impact are noted. International partnerships that build research capacity and expertise offer particular promise, an example being Reavley and Jorm's mental health literacy work.

Each chapter is a valuable resource in its own right but we would also highlight some important cross-cutting themes that emerge.

Equity

The importance of balancing population-level work with targeted initiatives with vulnerable groups must be considered at the outset of programmes. Contemporary public health approaches to mental health often focus upon concepts of health gain using population-based initiatives, exemplified by the use of social marketing models built on the notion of individual agency and responsibility (Quinn et al. 2011b). However, these universal approaches can fail to recognize or respond to inequalities and there has been an increasing recognition that there needs to be more of a focus on health equity rather than simply population health gain (The Marmot Review, Marmot 2010). The importance of taking action in tackling inequalities in mental health and illness emerges as a key argument throughout the book for example in the chapters by Hanlon and Carlisle, Mathieson et al. and Maxwell.

Determinants

We would highlight the need to maintain a focus on social determinants within (Pickett and Wilkinson) and between both higher- and lower-income countries (Petersen and Lund). Here, linking mental health to anti-poverty measures is critical. There is a strong body of evidence that lower socioeconomic status is associated with poorer mental health, with the poorest section of the population twice as likely to be at risk of developing mental health problems as those on average incomes (Fryers et al. 2003; Palmer et al. 2003). This extends beyond socio-economic factors to addressing mental health inequities that are linked to dimensions of identity including gender, sexuality, disability and ethnicity (Quinn and Knifton 2012) that can be manifested as trauma, discrimination/exclusion, abuse and stress. Early years are critical (Barlow). But although this wider social challenge can seem beyond the sphere of influence of activists and practitioners in public mental health, we can play an important role. We can ensure that activities to reduce stigma or promote recovery reach out to all communities and that programmes that support families, schools and elderly people are focused upon communities that are most vulnerable. Work and employment, which Jané-Llopis and Cooper highlight as a major factor in promoting mental health and wellbeing, is also the main way of redistributing wealth in societies and our attention should not just be upon improving the conditions of work but ensuring that employers recruit from areas of low employment. Finally, we must remember that people with long-term mental health problems can be a marginalized group and we should advocate for continued investment in progressive services as highlighted by Byrne for early intervention and Nash for physical health. And this should be invested to a greater extent in areas of need, in line with the notion of proportionate universalism (Marmot 2010).

Empowering individuals and communities

A further theme that complements rather than competes with action on determinants is empowerment. We see this in several ways in the book, for example Stewart-Brown and Reavley and Jorm discuss the empowerment of individuals at a population level whereas Rüsch and Corrigan and O'Hagan explore empowerment as a route to equality and recovery for people with mental health problems. We can see how empowerment is important in population programmes, for example through mental health literacy, in relation to parenting skills and school programmes, where individuals are enabled to have the confidence and skills to improve the mental health of themselves and others. But beyond this we see that empowering communities, through community development approaches and asset-based work, can be an approach that links macro- and micro-level interventions (Quinn 2010). Community features heavily throughout, whether in the importance of supportive communities in Cattan's discussion on reducing isolation in later life or Rüsch and Corrigan's focus upon exclusion/acceptance, through to communities such as schools (Mulloy and Weist) and workplaces that have an equally significant impact on mental health and wellbeing. With long-term trends pointing towards greater social isolation (Putnam 2000) there is a strong argument for social connectedness and loneliness being a major priority for future public mental health. Interestingly, other than the chapters on early years and later life, there is modest attention given to the importance of family in the book, which should perhaps be a major focus of future work in this area, given that for most people it forms our immediate and most significant community and social network.

Communities of practice

We see throughout the book, and also in drawing upon our own practice and experience in this area, that there is a need to develop new models of leadership and action in public mental health. This is necessary to respond to the complexity and the scale of the challenges that we face. We have seen that it is important to draw together different disciplines and perspectives, to shape policy across different domains, and to develop and evaluate programmes that work at individual, local and national levels simultaneously. This means that public mental health is complex and compromises are necessary. To add to this challenge, many areas of public mental health have developed in silos over the past decades. This is because the agenda has been driven by policy priorities, such as with suicide prevention activity, or advocacy by professional groups, such as with anti-stigma work, or through grassroots activism, as we have seen in the recovery movement. However, the chapters within the book illustrate how often these developments are interconnected and can be tackled more efficiently and effectively when they are brought together. This means that we need effective yet collaborative leadership. Such a model of leadership might on one day be setting targets for funders and on another be negotiating between groups with diverse perspectives and agendas. This can only be achieved, in our opinion, through communities of practice (Wenger 1998). Working at these different levels requires the orchestration of strong partnerships between policy makers, academics, service planners, practitioners, NGOs and communities. This model has the potential to maximize collaborative effort and encourage shared ownership, especially important in challenging economic times, and to stimulate and develop innovative approaches to public mental health. The importance of collaborations is seen throughout the chapters where non-health specialists are vital partners in reaching communities – for example parents (Barlow), schools (Mulloy and Weist), early intervention with adolescents (Byrne) or older people (Cattan).

International action

Finally, the book also begins to highlight the growing importance of fostering international connections in public mental health. This is partly about sharing learning but more fundamentally about the interconnectedness of local, national and global wellbeing – as highlighted by Hanlon and Carlisle in the opening chapter. The importance of an international focus can be seen throughout the book – in relation to resource-scarce countries in Petersen and Lund, in relation to suicide prevention by Beautrais and Larkin, and clearly in relation to workplace mental health in Jané–Llopis and Cooper. The recent development of a Global Movement for Mental Health (see www.globalmentalhealth.org) and the new WHO programme on Health Rights (see www.health-rights.org) highlight the importance of incorporating an understanding of global influences on mental health when defining priorities for policy and practice. In doing so, we need to ensure we do not simply import public mental health initiatives from higher- to lower-income countries but also consider what can be learned *by* higher-income countries, for example recognition of the role and value of older people within society or a greater emphasis upon community development approaches that build upon informal social networks. We must also recognize the significance of social, cultural and religious constructions of health (Knifton 2012).

References

Adelman, H.S. and Taylor, L. (2000) Promoting mental health in schools in the midst of school reform, *The Journal of School Health*, 70: 171–178.

Aked, J., Marks, N., Cordon, C. and Thompson, S. (2008) *Five Ways to Wellbeing*. London: Centre for Wellbeing, New Economics Foundation (www.nef.org.uk).

Albee, G.W. (1982) Preventing psychopathology and promoting human potential, *American Psychologist*, 37: 1043–1057.

Alinsky, S.D. (1972) *Rules for Radicals: a Pragmatic Primer for Realistic Radicals*. New York: Vintage Books.

Allbright, A.L. (2005) 2004 employment decisions under the ADA Title I – Survey update, *Mental and Physical Disability Law Reporter*, 29: 513–516.

Altamura, A.C., Dell'Osso, B., Vismara, S. and Mundo, E. (2008a) May duration of untreated illness influence the long-term course of major depressive disorder?, *European Psychiatry*, 23: 92–96.

Altamura, A.C., Dell'Osso, B., D'Urso, N., Russo, M., Fumagalli, S. and Mundo, E. (2008b) Duration of untreated illness as a predictor of treatment response and clinical course in generalized anxiety disorder, *CNS Spectrums*, 13: 415–422.

Altamura, A.C., Dell'Osso, B., Berlin, H.A., Buoli, M., Bassetti, R. and Mundo, E. (2010) Duration of untreated illness and suicide in bipolar disorder: a naturalistic study, *European Archives of Psychiatry and Clinical Neuroscience*, 260: 385–391.

Ambrose, M.G., Weist, M.D., Schaeffer, C., Nabors, L.A. and Hill, S. (2002) Evaluation and quality improvement in school mental health, in H.S. Ghuman, M.D. Weist and R.M. Sarles (eds) *Providing Mental Health Services to Youth Where They Are: School and Community-Based Approaches*: 95–112. New York: Brunner-Routledge.

American Academy of Pediatrics Committee on School Health (2004) Policy statement: School-based mental health services, *Pediatrics*, 113: 1839–1845.

Anderson, P., Jané-Llopis, E. and Cooper, C. (2011) The imperative of well-being, *Stress and Health*, 27: 353–355.

Andis, P., Cashman, J., Praschil, R., Oglesby, D., Adelman, H., Taylor, L. and Weist, M.D. (2002) A strategic and shared agenda to advance mental health in schools through family and system partnerships, *International Journal of Mental Health Promotion*, 4: 28–35.

Angermeyer, M.C. and Dietrich, S. (2006) Public beliefs about and attitudes towards people with mental illness: a review of population studies, *Acta Psychiatrica Scandinavica*, 113: 163–179.

Angermeyer, M.C. and Matschinger, H. (2005) Have there been any changes in the public's attitudes towards psychiatric treatment? Results from representative population surveys in Germany in the years 1990 and 2001, *Acta Psychiatrica Scandanavica*, 111: 68–73.

Angermeyer, M.C., Breier, P., Dietrich, S., Kenzine, D. and Matschinger, H. (2005) Public attitudes toward psychiatric treatment. An international comparison, *Social Psychiatry and Psychiatric Epidemiology*, 40: 855–864.

Angst, J., Gamma, A. and Endrass, J. (2003) Risk factors for the bipolar and depression spectra, *Acta Psychiatrica Scandanavica*, 418: 15–19.

Anthony, W. (1993) Recovery from mental illness: the guiding vision of the mental health service system in the 1990s, *Psychosocial Rehabilitation Journal*, 16: 11–23.

Anthony, W. (2000) A recovery-oriented service system: setting some system level standards, *Psychiatric Rehabilitation Journal*, 24: 159–168.

Antonovsky, A. (1979) *Health, Stress and Coping*. San Francisco: Jossey-Bass Publishers.

Arnstein, S. (1969) A ladder of community participation, *Journal of the American Planning Association*, 35: 216–224.

Australian Bureau of Statistics (2003) *National Health Survey, Mental Health, 2001*. Australian Bureau of Statistics.

Australian Social Inclusion Board (2008) *National Mental Health and Disability Consultation Findings*. Canberra: Australian Government.

Baicker, K., Cutler, D. and Song, Z. (2010) Workplace wellness programs can generate savings, *Health Affairs*, 29: 304–311.

Barlow, J., Schrader McMillan, A., Kirkpatrick, S., Ghate, D., Smith M. and Barnes, J. (2009) *Health-led Parenting interventions in Pregnancy and Early Years*, London: DCSF.

Barnett, W.S. (1995) Long-term effects of early childhood programs on cognitive and school outcomes, *The Future of Children*, 5: 25–50.

Barry, M.M. (2001) Promoting positive mental health: Theoretical frameworks for practice, *The International Journal of Mental Health Promotion*, 3: 25–34.

Barry, M.M. (2007) Researching the implementation of community mental health promotion programs, *Health Promotion Journal of Australia*, 18: 240–246.

Bartley, M. (ed) (2006) *Capability and Resilience: Beating the Odds*. London: ESRC Human Capability and Resilience Research Network London, UCL Department of Epidemiology and Public Health.

Battaglia, J., Coverdale, J.H. and Bushong, C.P. (1990) Evaluation of a Mental Illness Awareness Week program in public schools, *American Journal of Psychiatry*, 147: 324–329.

Battin-Pearson, S., Newcomb, M.D., Abbot, R.D., Hill, K.G., Catalano, R.F. and Hawkins, J.D. (2000) Predictors of early high school dropout: a test of five theories, *Journal of Educational Psychology*, 92: 568–582.

Bauman, Z. (1998) *Work, Consumerism and the New Poor*. Buckingham: Open University Press.

Bauman, Z. (2001) *The Individualized Society*. Cambridge: Polity Press.

Beautrais, A.L. (2005) National strategies for the reduction and prevention of suicide, *Crisis*, 26: 1–3.

Beautrais, A.L., Fergusson, D.M. and Horwood, L.J. (2006) Firearms legislation and reductions in firearm-related suicide deaths in New Zealand, *Australian and New Zealand Journal of Psychiatry*, 40: 253–259.

Beautrais, A.L., Gibb, S.J., Fergusson, D.M., Horwood, L.J. and Larkin, G.L. (2009) Removing bridge barriers stimulates suicides: an unfortunate natural experiment, *Australian and New Zealand Journal of Psychiatry*, 43: 495–497.

Bech, P. (2004) Measuring the dimensions of psychological general well-being by the WHO-5, *QoL Newsletter*, 32: 15–16.

Bechdolf, A., Wagner, M., Ruhrmann, S., Harrigan, S., Putzfeld, V., Pukrop, R., Brockhaus-Dumke, A., Berning, J., Janssen, B., Decker, P., Bottlender, R., Maurer, K., Möller, H., Gaebel, W., Häfner, H., Maier, W. and Klosterkötter, J. (2012) Preventing progression to first-episode psychosis in early initial prodromal states, *British Journal of Psychiatry*, 200: 22–29.

Beck, A.T., Ward, C. and Mendelson, M. (1961) Beck Depression Inventory (BDI), *Archives of General Psychiatry*, 4: 561–571.

Beck, A.T., Steer, R.A. and Brown, G.K. (1996) *Manual for the Beck Depression Inventory-II*. San Antonio, TX: Psychological Corporation.

Beck, U. (1992) *Risk Society: Towards a New Modernity*. New Delhi: Sage.

Beebe, B., Jaffe, J., Markese, S., Buck, K., Chen, H., Cohen, P., Bahrick, L., Andrews, H. and Feldstein, S. (2010) The origins of 12-month attachment: a microanalysis of 4-month mother-infant interaction, *Attachment and Human Development*, 12: 3–141.

Bell, C.C., Bhana, A., Petersen, I., McKay, M.M., Gibbons. R., Bannon, W. and Amatya, A. (2008) Building protective factors to offset sexually risky behaviors among black youths: a randomized control trial, *Journal of the National Medical Association*, 100: 936–944.

Benoit, D., Parker, K. and Zeanah, C. (1997) Mothers' representations of their infants assessed pre-natally: stability and association with infants' attachment classifications, *Journal of Child Psychology, Psychiatry, and Allied Disciplines*, 38: 307–313.

Bergner, S., Monk, C. and Wagner, E.A. (2008) Dyadic intervention during pregnancy? Treating pregnant women and possibly reaching the future baby, *Infant Mental Health Journal*, 29: 399–419.

Berlin, L.J., Cassidy, J. and Appleyard, K. (2008) The influence of early attachments on other relationships, in J. Cassidy and P.R. Shaver (eds), *Handbook of Attachment: Theory, Research and Clinical Applications*. New York: Guilford Press.

Bertolote, J. and McGorry, P. (2005) Early intervention and recovery for young people with early psychosis: consensus statement (on behalf of the World Health Organization and the International Early Psychosis Association), *British Journal of Psychiatry*, 187: 116–119.

Bhana, A. (2010) Middle childhood and pre-adolescence, in I. Petersen, A. Petersen, A. Bhana, A.J. Flisher, L. Swartz and L. Richter (eds), *Promoting Mental Health in Scarce-Resource Contexts. Emerging Evidence and Practice*. Cape Town: HSRC Press.

Bhana, A. and Govender, A. (2010) Evaluating interventions, in I. Petersen, A. Petersen, A. Bhana, A.J. Flisher, L. Swartz, and L. Richter (eds), *Promoting Mental Health in Scarce-Resource Contexts. Emerging Evidence and Practice*. Cape Town: HSRC Press.

Bloom, D.E., Cafiero, E.T., Jané-Llopis, E., Abrahams-Gessel, S., Bloom, L.R., Fathima, S. and Weinstein, C. (2011) *The Global Economic Burden of Non-Communicable Diseases*. Geneva: World Economic Forum.

Blum, R.W., McNeely, C. and Rinehart, P.M. (2002) *Improving the Odds: The Untapped Power of Schools to Improve the Health of Teens*. Minneapolis, MN: Center for Adolescent Health and Development, University of Minnesota.

Bodenhausen, G.V. and Richeson, J.A. (2010) Prejudice, stereotyping, and discrimination, in R.F. Baumeister and E.J. Finkel (eds), *Advanced Social Psychology* (pp. 341–384). Oxford: Oxford University Press.

Boersma, K. and Linton, S.J. (2005) Screening to identify patients at risk: profiles of psychological risk factors for early intervention, *Clinical Journal of Pain*, 21: 38–43.

Borges, G., Nock, M.K., Haro Abad, J.M., Hwang, I., Sampson, N.A., Alonso, J., Andrade, L.H., Angermeyer, M.C., Beautrais, A., Bromet, E., Bruffaerts, R., de Girolamo, G., Florescu, S., Gureje, O., Hu, C., Karam, E.G., Kovess-Masfety, V., Lee, S., Levinson, D., Medina-Mora, M.E., Ormel, J., Posada-Villa, J., Sagar, R., Tomov, T., Uda, H., Williams D.R. and Kessler, R.C. (2010) Twelve-month prevalence of and risk factors for suicide attempts in the World Health Organization World Mental Health Surveys, *Journal of Clinical Psychiatry*, 71: 1617–1628.

Bourdieu, P. (1984) *Distinction: A Social Critique of the Judgement of Taste*. London: Routledge.

Bower, P., Gilbody, S.M., Richards, D., Fletcher, J. and Sutton, A. (2006) Collaborative care for depression in primary care. Making sense of a complex intervention: systematic review and meta-regression, *British Journal of Psychiatry*, 189: 484–493.

Bowlby, J. (1969) *Attachment and Loss: Volume I: Attachment*. New York: Basic Books.

Bowlby, J. (1973) *Attachment and Loss: Volume II: Separation, Anxiety and Anger*. New York: Basic Books.

Bowlby, J. (1979) *The Making and Breaking of Affectional Bonds*. London: Tavistock.

Bowling, A. and Gabriel, Z. (2007) Lay theories of quality of life in older age, *Ageing and Society*, 27: 827–848.

Brandt, R. (2009) Putting mental health on the agenda for HIV+ women: a review of evidence from sub-Saharan Africa, *Women Health*, 49: 215–228.

Brickman, P., Coates, D. and Janoff-Bulman, R. (1978) Lottery winners and accident victims: is happiness relative? *Journal of Personal and Social Psychology*, 36: 917–927.

Brown, M.M. and Grumet, J.G. (2009) School-based suicide prevention with African American youth in an urban setting, *Professional Psychology: Research and Practice*, 40: 111–117.

Bruce, M.L. and Hoff, R.A. (1994) Social and physical health risk factors for first-onset major depressive disorder in a community sample, *Social Psychiatry and Psychiatric Epidemiology*, 29: 165–171.

Bruns, E.J., Walrath, C., Glass-Siegal, M. and Weist, M.D. (2004) School-based mental health services in Baltimore: association with school climate and special education referrals, *Behavior Modification*, 28: 491–512.

Buist-Bouwman, M.A., de Graaf, R., Vollebergh, W.A.M. and Ormel, J. (2005) Comorbidity of physical and mental disorders and the effect on work-loss days, *Acta Psychiatrica Scandinavica*, 111: 436–443.

Burgher, M.S., Rasmussen, V.B. and Rivett, D. (1999) *The European Network of Health Promoting Schools*. IPC, Copenhagen: The Alliance of Education and Health.

Burke, R.W. and Paternite, C.E. (2007) Teacher engagement in expanded school mental health, in S.W. Evans, M.D. Weist and N. Zewelanji (eds), *Advances in School-Based Mental Health Interventions: Best Practices and Program Models, Vol. II* (pp. 1–15). Kingston, NJ: Civic Research Institute.

Burns, B.J., Costello, E.J., Angold, A., Tweed, D., Stangl, D., Farmer, E.M. and Erkanli, A. (1995) Children's mental health service use across service sectors, *Health Affairs*, 14, 147–159.

Burns, J.R. and Rapee, R.M. (2006) Adolescent mental health literacy: young people's knowledge of depression and help seeking, *Journal of Adolescence*, 29: 225–239.

Bushe, C. and Holt, R. (2004) Prevalence of diabetes and impaired glucose tolerance in patients with schizophrenia, *British Journal of Psychiatry*, 184: 67–71.

Byrne, P. (2007) Managing the acute psychotic episode, *British Medical Journal*, 334: 686–692.

Cafaro, P. (2001) Economic consumption, pleasure, and the good life, *Journal of Social Philosophy*, 32: 471–486.

Cameron, I.M., Crawford, J.R., Lawton, K. and Reid, I.C. (2008). Psychometric comparison of PHQ-9 and HADS for measuring depression severity in primary care, *British Journal of General Practice*, 58: 32–36.

Capella-McDonnall, M.E. (2005) The effects of single and dual sensory loss on symptoms of depression in the elderly, *International Journal of Geriatric Psychiatry*, 20: 855–861.

Carlisle, S. and Hanlon, P. (2007) The complex territory of well-being: contestable evidence, contentious theories and speculative conclusions, *Journal of Public Mental Health*, 6: 8–13.

Carlisle, S. and Hanlon, P. (2008) 'Wellbeing' as a focus for public health? A critique and defence, *Critical Public Health*, 18: 263–270.

Carlisle, S., Snooks, H., Evans, A. and Cohen, D. (2007) Evaluation, evidence and learning in community-based action research, in S. Cropper, A. Porter, G. Williams, S. Carlisle, R. Moore, M. O'Neill, C. Roberts, H. Snooks (eds), *Community Health and Wellbeing: Action Research on Health Inequalities*. Bristol: Policy Press.

Carlisle, S., Henderson, G. and Hanlon, P. (2009) 'Wellbeing': a collateral casualty of modernity? *Social Science and Medicine*, 69: 1556–1560.

Carpiano, R.M. (2006) Toward a neighborhood resource-based theory of social capital for health: can Bourdieu and sociology help? *Social Science and Medicine*, 62: 165–175.

Catalano, R.F., Haggerty, K.P., Oesterle, S., Fleming, C.B. and Hawkins, J.D. (2004) The importance of bonding to school for healthy development: findings from the Social Development Research Group, *Journal of School Health*, 74: 252–261.

Cattan, M., White, M., Bond, J. and Learmonth, A. (2005) Preventing social isolation and loneliness among older people: a systematic review of health promotion interventions, *Ageing and Society*, 25: 41–67.

Cattan, M., Hughes, S., Fylan, F., Kime, N. and Giuntoli, G. (2010) *The Needs of Frail Older People with Sight Loss. (Occasional paper No 29)*. London: Thomas Pocklington Trust.

Cattan, M., Hobbs, E. and Hardill, I. (2011a) Improving quality of life in ageing populations: What can volunteering do?, *Maturitas*, 70: 328–332.

Cattan, M., Kime, N. and Bagnall, A.M. (2011b) The use of telephone befriending in low level support for socially isolated older people – an evaluation, *Health and Social Care in the Community*, 19: 198–206.

Center for Disease Control and Prevention (2007) *Compressed Mortality Files 1999–2006*. Atlanta: Center for Disease Control and Prevention. Available at http://wonder.cdc.gov/mortsql.html (accessed 23 August 2012).

Centre for Economic Performance's Mental Health Policy Group (2006) *The Depression Report: A New Deal for Depression and Anxiety Disorders*. London: London School of Economics.

Centre for Mental Health (2011) The Economic and Social Costs of Mental Health Problems in 2009/10. London: Centre for Mental Health. Available at www.centreformentalhealth.org.uk (accessed 28 August 2012).

Chamberlin, J. (1978) *On our Own: Patient-Controlled Alternatives to the Mental Health System*. New York: Hawthorn Books, Inc.

Chambers, D.A., Pearson, J.L., Lubell, K., Brandon, S., O'Brien, K. and Zinn, J. (2005) The science of public messages for suicide prevention: a workshop summary, *Suicide and Life Threatening Behaviour*, 35: 134–145.

Chambers, R. (1997) *Whose Reality Counts?* London: Intermediate Technology.

Chandola, T., Ferrie, J., Sacker, A. and Marmot, M. (2007) Social inequalities in self reported health in early old age: follow-up of prospective cohort study, *British Medical Journal*, 334: 990–994.

Chang, C.-K., Hayes, R.D., Perera, G., Broadbent, M.T.M., Fernandes, A.C., Lee, W.E., Hotopf, M. and Stewart, R. (2011) Life expectancy at birth for people with serious mental illness and other major disorders from a secondary mental health care case register in London, *PLoS One*, 6, 5: e19590.

Charuvastra, A. and Cloitre, M. (2008) Social bonds and posttraumatic stress disorder, *Annual Review of Psychology*, 59: 301–328.

Child and Adolescent Health Measurement Initiative (2006) *National Survey of Children's Health, Data Resource Center on Child and Adolescent Health. Child and Adolescent Health Measurement Initiative*. Portland: CAHMI. Available at www.childhealthdata.org/learn/NSCH (accessed 23 August 2012).

Chisolm, D., Flisher, A.J., Lund, C., Patel, V., Saxena, S., Thornicroft, G. and Tomlinson, M. (2007) Scale up services for mental disorders: a call for action, *Lancet*, 370: 1241–1252.

Chorpita, B.F. and Daleiden, E.L. (2007) *2007 Biennial Report: Effective Psychosocial Intervention for Youth with Behavioral and Emotional Needs*. Hawaii: Child and Mental Health Division, Hawaii Department of Health.

Chorpita, B.F. and Daleiden, E.L. (2010) Building evidence-based systems in children's mental health, in A.E. Kazdin and J.R. Weisz (eds), *Evidence-Based Psychotherapies for Children and Adolescents* (pp. 482–499). New York: Oxford.

Christensen, H., Griffiths, K.M. and Jorm, A.F. (2004) Delivering interventions for depression by using the internet: randomised controlled trial, *British Medical Journal*, 328: 265.

Christensen, H., Leach, L.S., Barney, L., MacKinnon, A.J. and Griffiths, K.M. (2006) The effect of web based depression interventions on self reported help seeking: randomised controlled trial, *BMC Psychiatry*, 6: 13.

Churchill, R., Hunot, V., Corney, R., Knapp, M., McGuire, H., Tylee, A. and Wessley, S. (2001) A systematic review of controlled trials of the effectiveness and cost-effectiveness of brief psychological treatments for depression, *Health Technology Assessment*, 5: 1–173.

Cipriani, A., Furukawa, T.A., Salanti, G., Geddes, J.R., Higgins, J.P., Churchill, R., Watanabe, N., Nakagawa, A., Omori, I.M., McGuire, H., Tansella, M. and Barbui, C. (2009) Comparative efficacy and acceptability of 12 new-generation antidepressants, *Lancet*, 373: 746–758.

Citrome, L. and Vreeland, B. (2009) Obesity and mental illness, in J. Thakore and B.E. Leonard (eds), *Metabolic Effects of Psychotropic Drugs Modern Trends in Pharmacopsychiatry* (pp. 25–46). Basel: Karger.

Claassen, C.A. and Larkin, G.L. (2005) Occult suicidality in an emergency department population, *British Journal of Psychiatry*, 186: 352–353.

Clarke, A., Friede, T., Putz, R., Ashdown, J., Martin, S., Blake, A., Adi, Y., Parkinson, J., Flynn, P., Platt, S. and Stewart-Brown, S. (2011). Warwick-Edinburgh Mental Well-being Scale (WEMWBS): mixed methods assessment of validity and reliability in teenage school students in England and Scotland, *BMC Public Health*, 11: 487.

Clow, A. and Aitchison, L. (2009) Keeping active, in M. Cattan (ed), *Mental Health and Well-being in Later Life* (pp.112–135). Maidenhead: Open University Press/McGraw-Hill.

Cohen, N., Muir, E., Lojkasek, M., Muir, R., Parker, C.J., Barwick, M. and Brown, M. (1999) Watch, wait and wonder: testing the effectiveness of a new approach to mother-infant psychotherapy, *Infant Mental Health Journal*, 20: 429–451.

Cohen, N.J., Loikasek, M., Muir, E., Muir, R. and Parker, C.J. (2002) Six-month follow-up of two mother-infant psychotherapies: convergence of therapeutic outcomes, *Infant Mental Health Journal*, 23: 4361–4380.

Collins, P.Y., Patel, V., Joestl, S.S., March, D., Insel, T.R., Daar, A.S.; Scientific Advisory Board and the Executive Committee of the Grand Challenges on Global Mental Health, Anderson, W., Dhansay, M.A., Phillips, A., Shurin, S., Walport, M., Ewart, W., Savill, S.J., Bordin, I.A., Costello, E.J., Durkin, M., Fairburn, C., Glass, R.I., Hall, W., Huang, Y., Hyman, S.E., Jamison, K., Kaaya, S., Kapur, S., Kleinman, A., Ogunniyi, A., Otero-Ojeda, A., Poo, M.M., Ravindranath, V., Sahakian, B.J., Saxena, S., Singer, P.A. and Stein, D.J. (2011) Grand challenges in global mental health, *Nature*, 475: 27–30.

Colton, C.W. and Manderscheid, R.W. (2006) Congruencies in increased mortality rates, years of potential life lost, and causes of death among public mental health clients in eight states, *Preventing Chronic Disease*, 3: A42.

Commission on Social Determinants of Health (2008) *Closing the Gap in a Generation: Health Equity Through Action on the Social Determinants of Health. Final Report of the Commission on Social Determinants of Health*. Geneva: WHO.

Compagni, A., Adams, N. and Daniels, A. (2006) *International Pathways to Mental Health System Transformation: Strategies and Challenges*. Sacramento, CA: California Institute for Mental Health.

Cooper, C.L. and Dewe, P. (2008) Well-being – absenteeism, presenteeism, costs and challenges, *Occupational Medicine*, 58: 522–524.

Cooper, C.L., Field, J., Goswami, U., Jenkins, R. and Sahakian, B. (2010) *Mental Capital and Wellbeing*. Oxford: Wiley-Blackwell.

Cooper, P.J., Tomlinson, M., Swartz, I., Landman, M., Molteno, C., Stein, A., McPherson, K. and Murray, I. (2009) Improving quality of mother-infant relationship and infant attachment in socioeconomically deprived community in South Africa: randomised controlled trial, *British Medical Journal*, 338: b974.

Coote, A., Allen, J. and Woodhead, D. (2004) *Finding Out What Works: Building Knowledge About Complex, Community-Based Initiatives. Policy Paper November 2004*. London: King's Fund.

Corrigan, P.W. (2005) *On the Stigma of Mental Illness: Practical Strategies for Research and Social Change*. Washington DC: American Psychological Association.

Corrigan, P.W. (2011) Strategic Stigma Change (SSC): five principles for social marketing campaigns meant to erase the prejudice and discrimination of mental illness, *Psychiatric Services*, 62: 824–826.

Corrigan, P.W. and Penn, D.L. (1999) Lessons from social psychology on discrediting psychiatric stigma, *American Psychologist*, 54: 765–776.

Corrigan, P.W. and Rüsch, N. (2002) Mental illness stereotypes and clinical care: do people avoid treatment because of stigma?, *Psychiatric Rehabilitation Skills*, 6: 312–334.

Corrigan, P.W. and Shapiro, J.R. (2010) Measuring the impact of programs that challenge the public stigma of mental illness, *Clinical Psychology Review*, 30: 907–922.

Corrigan, P.W., Markowitz, F.E. and Watson, A.C. (2004) Structural levels of mental illness stigma and discrimination, *Schizophrenia Bulletin*, 30: 481–491.

Corrigan, P.W. Watson, A.C., Heyrman, M.L., Warpinski, A., Gracia, G., Slopen, N. and Hall, L.L. (2005) Structural stigma in state legislation, *Psychiatric Services*, 56: 557–563.

Corrigan, P.W., Larson, J.E. and Rüsch, N. (2009) Self-stigma and the 'why try' effect: Impact on life goals and evidence-based practices, *World Psychiatry*, 8: 75–81.

Corrigan, P.W., Roe, D. and Tsang, H.W. (2011). *Challenging the Stigma of Mental Illness: Lessons for Therapists and Advocates*. Chichester: Wiley-Blackwell.

Cowen, M. (2009) Early-onset mental health disorders linked to non-completion of education, *British Journal of Psychiatry*, 194: 411–417.

Coyne, J., Palmer, S. and Sullivan, P. (2003) Screening for depression in adults, *Annals of Internal Medicine*, 138: 767–768.

Craig, T. (2006) What is psychiatric rehabilitation?, in G. Roberts, S. Davenport, F. Holloway and T. Tattan (eds), *Enabling Recovery: The Principles and Practice of Psychiatric Rehabilitation*. London: Gaskell.

Croghan, T.W., Tomlin, M., Pescosolido, B.A., Schnittker, J., Martin, J., Lubell, K. and Swindle, R. (2003) American attitudes toward and willingness to use psychiatric medications, *Journal of Nervous and Mental Disease*, 191: 166–174.

Csikszentmihalyi, M. (2004) What we must accomplish in the coming decades, *Zygon*, 39: 359–366.

Csikszentmihalyi, M. and Csikszentmihalyi, I.S. (1988) *Optimal Experience: Psychological Studies of Flow in Consciousness*. New York: Cambridge University Press.

Cuijpers, P., van Straten, A., van Schaik, A. and Andersson, G. (2009) Psychological treatment of depression in primary care: a meta-analysis, *British Journal of General Practice*, 59: 51–60.

Cusack, J., Deane, F.P., Wilson, C.J. and Ciarocchi, J. (2004) Who influences men to go to therapy? Reports from men attending psychological services, *International Journal for the Advancement of Counselling*, 26: 271–283.

Czabała, C., Charzyńska, K. and Mroziak, B. (2011) Psychosocial interventions in workplace mental health promotion – an overview, *Health Promotion International*, 26: 70–84.

Dahlberg, K.M., Waern, M. and Runeson, B. (2008) Mental health literacy and attitudes in a Swedish community sample – investigating the role of personal experience of mental health care, *BMC Public Health*, 8: 8.

Davidson, L., Tondora, J. and O'Connell, M. (2007) Creating a recovery-oriented system of behavioral health care: moving from concept to reality, *Psychiatric Rehabilitation Journal*, 31: 23–31.

Day, R. (2008) Local environments and older people's health: dimensions from a comparative qualitative study in Scotland, *Health and Place*, 14: 299–312.

de Botton, A. (2004) *Status Anxiety*. Melbourne: Hamish Hamilton.

De Hert, M., Correll, U.C., Bobes, J., Cetkovich-Bakmas, M., Cohen, D., Asai, I., Detraux, J., Gautam, S., Möller, H.-J., Ndetei, D., Newcomer, J.W., Uwakwe, J. and Leucht, S. (2011) WPA Educational Module: physical illness in patients with severe mental disorders, *World Psychiatry*, 10: 52–77.

De Wolff, M.S. and van Ijzendoorn, M.H. (1997) Sensitivity and attachment: a meta-analysis on parental antecedents of infant attachment, *Child Development*, 68: 571–591.

Deegan, P. (1988) Recovery: the lived experience of rehabilitation, *Psychosocial Rehabilitation Journal*, 9: 11–19.

Deegan, P. (1990) *How Recovery Begins.* Lawrence, MA: National Empowerment Center.

Deegan, P. (1992) *Recovery, Rehabilitation and the Conspiracy of Hope.* Lawrence, MA: National Empowerment Center.

Demyttenaere, K., Bruffaerts, R., Posada-Villa, J., Gasquet, I., Kovess, V., Lepine, J.P. Angermeyer, M.C., Bernert, S., de Girolamo, G., Morosini, P., Polidori, G., Kikkawa, T., Kawakami, N., Ono, Y., Takeshima, T., Uda, H., Karam, E.G., Fayyad, J.A., Karam, A.N., Mneimneh, Z.N., Medina-Mora, M.E., Borges, G., Lara, C., de Graaf, R., Ormel, J., Gureje, O., Shen, Y., Huang, Y., Zhang, M., Alonso, J., Haro, J.M., Vilagut, G., Bromet, E.J., Gluzman, S., Webb, C., Kessler, R.C., Merikangas, K.R., Anthony, J.C., Von Korff, M.R., Wang, P.S., Brugha, T.S., Aguilar-Gaxiola, S., Lee, S., Heeringa, S., Pennell, B.E., Zaslavsky, A.M., Ustun, T.B., Chatterji, S.; WHO World Mental Health Survey Consortium. (2004) Prevalence, severity, and unmet need for treatment of mental disorders in the World Health Organization World Mental Health Surveys, *Journal of the American Medical Association*, 291: 2581–2590.

Department for Communities and Local Government (2010) *Evaluation of the National Strategy for Neighbourhood Renewal.* London: Communities and Local Government Publishing.

Department for Environment, Food and Rural Affairs (2011) *Life Satisfaction and other Measures of Wellbeing in England 2007–2011.* London: DEFRA.

Department of Health (2001a) *Treatment Choice in Psychological Therapies and Counselling: Evidence-Based Clinical Practice Guideline.* London: Stationery Office.

Department of Health (2001b) *Making it Happen: A Guide to Delivering Mental Health Promotion.* Department of Health: London.

Department of Health (2001c) *Mental Health Policy Implementation Guidance.* London: Department of Health Publications. Available at http://www.dh.gov.uk/en/Publicationsandstatistics/Publications/PublicationsPolicyAndGuidance/DH_4009350 (accessed 25 August 2012).

Department of Health (2008) *Improving Access to Psychological Therapies Implementation Plan.* Department of Health: London.

Department of Health (2009) *Healthy Child Programme: Pregnancy and the First Five Years of Life.* London: Department of Health.

Department of Health (2010a) *Healthy Lives Healthy People,* London: Department of Health.

Department of Health (2010b) *Confident Communities Brighter Futures: A Framework for Developing Well-being.* London: Department of Health.

Department of Health (2011a) *No Health without Mental Health: A Cross-Government Mental Health Outcomes Strategy for People of All Ages.* London: Department of Health.

Department of Health (2011b) *Quality and Outcomes Framework Guidance.* Department of Health: London.

Dew, M.A., Bromet, E.J., Schulberg, H.C., Parkinson, D.K. and Curtis, E.C. (1991) Factors affecting service utilization for depression in a white collar population, *Social Psychiatry and Psychiatric Epidemiology*, 26: 230–237.

Dewa, C.S., McDaid, D. and Ettner, S.L. (2007) An international perspective on worker mental health problems: who bears the burden and how are costs addressed?, *Canadian Journal of Psychiatry*, 52: 346–356.

Dewe, P. and Kompier, M. (2008) *Foresight Mental Capital and Wellbeing Project. Wellbeing and Work: Future Challenges.* London: The Government Office for Science.

Dey, A., Schiller, J. and Tai, D. (2004) Summary health statistics for U.S. children: National Health Interview Survey, 2002. National Center for Health Statistics, *Vital Health Statistics*, 10: 221.

Diener, E. (1984) Subjective well-being, *Psychological Bulletin*, 95: 542–575.

Diener, E., Emmons, R.A., Larsen, R.J. and Griffin, S. (1985) The satisfaction with life scale, *Journal of Personality Assessment*, 49: 71–75.

Diener, E. and Seligman, M.E. (2002) Very happy people, *Psychological Science*, 13(1): 81–84.

Diener, E., Wirtz, D., Tov, W., Kim-Prieto, C., Choi, D., Oishi, S. and Biswas-Diener, R. (2009) New measures of well-being: flourishing and positive and negative feelings, *Social Indicators Research*, 39: 247–266.

Dietrich, S., Mergl, R., Freudenberg, P., Althaus, D. and Hegerl, U. (2009) Impact of a campaign on the public's attitudes towards depression, *Health Education Research*, 25: 135–150.

Disability Rights Commission (2005) *Equal Treatment: Closing the Gap. Interim Report of a Formal Investigation into Health Inequalities.* Stratford upon Avon: Disability Rights Commission.

Dixon, L., Postrado, L., Delahanty. J., Fischer, P.J. and Lehman, A. (1999) The association of medical co morbidity in schizophrenia with poor physical health, *Journal of Nervous and Mental Disease*, 187: 496–502.

Donker, T., Griffiths, K.M., Cuijpers, P. and Christensen, H. (2009) Psychoeducation for depression, anxiety and psychological distress: a meta-analysis, *BMC Medicine*, 7: 79.

Donnellan, C. (2004) *Mental Wellbeing.* Cambridge: Independence Educational Publishers.

Dovidio, J.F. and Gaertner, S.L. (2010) Intergroup bias, in S.T. Fiske, D. Gilbert and G. Lindzey (eds), *Handbook of Social Psychology*, 5th edn (pp. 1084–1121). New York: Wiley.

Dowrick, C., Leydon, G.M., McBride, A., Howe, A., Burgess, H., Clarke, P., Maisey, S. and Kendrick, T. (2009) Patients' and doctors' views on depression severity questionnaires incentivised in UK quality and outcomes framework: qualitative study, *British Medical Journal*, 19: 338.

Druss, B.G. (2007) Improving medical care for persons with serious mental illness: challenges and solutions, *Journal of Clinical Psychiatry*, 68: 40–44.

Dumesnil, H. and Verger, P. (2009) Public awareness campaigns about depression and suicide: a review, *Psychiatric Services*, 60: 1203–1213.

Dunham, K. (2004) Young adults' support strategies when peers disclose suicidal intent, *Suicide and Life Threatening Behaviour*, 34: 56–65.

Dunion, L. and Gordon, L. (2005) Tackling the attitude problem. The achievements to date of Scotland's 'See Me' anti-stigma campaign, *Mental Health Today*, 22–25.

Durie, M. (2004) Indigeneity, and the promotion of positive mental health, *MindNet, Issue 2*. Auckland: Mental Health Foundation.

Durkin, M. (2002) The epidemiology of developmental disabilities in low-income countries, *Mental Retardation and Developmental Disabilities Research Reviews*, 8: 206–211.

Easterlin, R.A. (1974) Does economic growth improve the human lot?, in P.A. David and M.W. Reeder (eds), *Nations and Households in Economic Growth: Essays in Honor of Moses Abramovitz*. New York: Academic Press.

Eaton, S.B., Konner, M. and Shostak, M. (1988) Stone agers in the fast lane – chronic degenerative diseases in evolutionary perspective, *American Journal of Medicine*, 84: 739–749.

Eckersley, R. (2006) Is modern Western culture a health hazard? *International Journal of Epidemiology*, 35: 252–258.

Eddleston, M., Buckley, N.A., Gunnell, D., Dawson, A.H. and Konradsen, F. (2006) Identification of strategies to prevent death after pesticide self-poisoning using a Haddon Matrix, *Injury Prevention*, 12: 333–337.

Einarsen, S., Hoel, H., Zapf, D. and Cooper, C.L. (2011) *Bullying and Harassment in the Workplace*. Boca Raton, FL: CRC Press.

Ekman, P., Davidson, R.J., Ricard, M. and Callance, B.A. (2005) Buddhist and psychological perspectives on emotions and wellbeing, *Current Directions in Psychological Science*, 14: 59–63.

Esters, I.G., Cooker, P.G. and Ittenbach, R.F. (1998) Effects of a unit of instruction in mental health on rural adolescents' conceptions of mental illness and attitudes about seeking help, *Adolescence*, 33: 469–476.

European Union Public Health Information System (EUPHIX) (2009) *Determinants of Health*. Bilthoven: EUPHIX. Available at www.euphix.org (accessed 28 August 2012).

Evans, S.W. and Weist, M.D. (2004) Implementing empirically supported treatments in schools: what are we asking?, *Child and Family Psychology Review*, 7: 263–267.

Fairhurst, K. and Dowrick, C. (1996) Problems with recruitment in a randomized controlled trial of counselling in general practice: causes and implications, *Journal of Health Services Research and Policy*, 1: 77–80.

Featherstone, M. (1991) *Consumer Culture and Postmodernism*. London: Sage.

Fiscella, K. and Franks, P. (2000) Individual income, income inequality, health, and mortality: what are the relationships?, *Health Services Research*, 35: 307–318.

Fixsen, D., Naoom, S.F., Blasé, D.A., Friedman, R.M. and Wallace, F. (2005) *Implementation Research: A Synthesis of the Literature*. University of South Florida, Louis de la Parte Florida Mental Health Institute: The National Implementation Research Network (FMHI Publication #231).

Flay, B.R., Biglan, A., Boruch, R.F., Castro, F.G., Gottfredson, D., Kellam, S., Moscicki, E.K., Schinke, S., Valentine, J.C. and Ji, P. (2005) Standards of evidence: criteria for efficacy, effectiveness and dissemination, *Prevention Science*, 6: 151–175.

Fletcher, A., Evans, J. and Smeethm, L. (2008) *Impact of Sight Loss in Older People in Britain (Occasional Paper 19)*. London: Thomas Pocklington Trust.

Flisher, A.J. and Gevers, A. (2010) Adolescence, in I. Petersen, A. Petersen, A. Bhana, A.J. Flisher, L. Swartz and L. Richter (eds), *Promoting Mental Health in Scarce-Resource Contexts. Emerging Evidence and Practice*. Cape Town: HSRC Press.

Focus on Mental Health (2001) *An Uphill Struggle: Poverty and Mental Health. Final Report of the Focus on Mental Health Work Programme 2000/2001.* London: Mental Health Foundation.

Foster, S., Rollefson, M., Doksum, T., Noonan, D. and Robinson, G. (2005) *School Mental Health Services in the United States, 2002–2003.* DHHS Pub. No. (SMA) 05–4068. Rockville, MD: Center for Mental Health Services, Substance Abuse and Mental Health Services Administration.

Fournier, J.C., DeRubeis, R.J., Hollon, S.D., Dimidjian, S., Amsterdam, J.D., Shelton, R.C. and Fawcett, J. (2010) Antidepressant drug effects and depression severity: a patient-level meta-analysis, *Journal of the American Medical Association*, 303: 47–53.

Fraley, R.C. (2002) Attachment stability from infancy to adulthood: meta-analysis and dynamic modelling of developmental mechanisms, *Personality and Social Psychology Review*, 6: 123–151.

Fraley, R.C. and Waller, N.G. (1998) Adult attachment patterns: a test of the typological model, in J.A. Simpson and W.S. Rholes (eds), *Attachment Theory and Close Relationships.* New York: Guilford Press.

Frank, R.H. (1999) *Luxury Fever.* New York: Free Press.

Frayne, S.M., Halanych, J.H., Miller, D.R., Wang, F., Lin, H., Pogach, L., Sharkansky, E.J., Keane, T.M., Skinner, K.M., Rosen, C.S. and Berlowitz, D.R. (2005) Disparities in diabetes care: impact of mental illness, *Archives of Internal Medicine*, 165: 2631–2638.

Frederickson, B.L. (2005) The broaden-and-build theory of positive emotions, in F.A. Huppert, N. Baylis and B. Keverne (eds), *The Science of Wellbeing.* Oxford: Oxford University Press.

Freire, P. (1972) *Pedagogy of the Oppressed.* Harmondsworth: Penguin.

Frieden, T.R. (2010) A framework for public health action: the health impact pyramid, *American Journal of Public Health*, 100: 590–595.

Friedli, L. (2004) *Public Mental Health: The Art, Science and Politics of Creating a Mentally Healthy Society: A Four Nations Debate.* Conference in Edinburgh, October.

Friedli, L. (2009) *Mental Health, Resilience and Inequalities.* Copenhagen: WHO Regional Office for Europe.

Fryers, T., Melzer, D. and Jenkins, R. (2003) Social inequalities and the common mental disorders: a systematic review of the evidence, *Social Psychiatry and Psychiatric Epidemiology*, 38: 229–237.

Future Vision Coalition (2008) *A New Vision for Mental Health: Discussion Paper.* London: Future Vision Coalition.

Gajalakshmi, V. and Peto, R. (2007) Suicide rates in rural Tamil Nadu, South India: verbal autopsy of 39,000 deaths in 1997–98, *International Journal of Epidemiology*, 36: 203–207.

Gartlehner, G., Gaynes, B.N., Hansen, R.A., Thaler, K., Lux, L., Van Noord, M., Mager, U., Thieda, P., Gaynes, B.N., Wilkins, T., Strobelberger, M., Lloyd, S., Reichenpfader, U. and Lohr, K.N. (2008) Comparative benefits and harms of second-generation antidepressants for treating major depressive disorder, *Annals of Internal Medicine*, 149: 734–750.

Gawronski, B. and Bodenhausen, G.V. (2006) Associative and propositional processes in evaluation: an integrative review of implicit and explicit attitude change, *Psychological Bulletin*, 132: 692–731.

Gaziano, T.A., Bitton, A., Anand, S., Abrahams-Gessel, S. and Murphy, A. (2010) Growing epidemic of coronary heart disease in low- and middle-income countries, *Current Problems in Cardiology*, 35: 72–115.

Gergely, G. and Watson, J. (1996) The social biofeedback model of parental affect-mirroring, *International Journal of Psycho-Analysis*, 77: 118–121.

GHK (2010) *Volunteering in the European Union.* London: GHK.

Giannakouris, K. (2008) *Population and Social Conditions.* Luxembourg: Eurostat.

Gibson, M., Petticrew, M., Bambra, C., Sowden, S.J., Wright, K.E. and Whitehead, M. (2011) Housing and health inequalities: a synthesis of systematic reviews of interventions aimed at different pathways linking housing and health, *Health and Place*, 17: 175–184.

Giddens, A. (1991) *Modernity and Self-Identity: Self And Society in the Late Modern Age.* Palo Alto, CA: Stanford University Press.

Gilbody, S., House, A.O. and Sheldon, T.A. (2005) Screening and case finding instruments for depression, *Cochrane Database of Systematic Reviews*, 4: CD002792.

Gilbody, S.M., Whitty, P.M., Grimshaw, J.M. and Thomas, R.E. (2003) Improving the detection and management of depression in primary care, *Quality and Safety in Health Care*, 12: 149–155.

Gilhooly, M. (2002) *Transport and Ageing: Extending Quality of Life for Older People Via Public and Private Transport.* Glasgow: Paisley University.

Giuntoli, G. and Cattan, M. (2010) *Constructing a Model to Guide Investment in Older People's Mental Capital, Mental Health and Wellbeing* (internal report). Leeds: Leeds Metropolitan University/Northumbria University.

Glaser, D. (2000) Child abuse and neglect and the brain – a review, *Journal of Child Psychology and Psychiatry*, 41: 97–116.

Goffman, E. (1963) *Stigma: Notes on the Management of Spoiled Identity*. London: Penguin.

Goldberg, D.P. and Williams, P. (1988) *A User's Guide to the General Health Questionnaire*. Windsor: NFER-Nelson.

Goldney, R.D., Dunn, K.I., Dal Grande, E., Crabb, S. and Taylor, A. (2009) Tracking depression-related mental health literacy across South Australia: a decade of change, *Australian and New Zealand Journal of Psychiatry*, 43: 476–483.

Gonder, P.O. and Hymes, D. (1994) *Improving School Climate and Culture: Critical Issues Report*. Arlington, VA: American Association of School Administrators.

Gonzalez, J.M., Alegria, M., Prihoda, T.J., Copeland, L.A. and Zeber, J.E. (2009) How the relationship of attitudes toward mental health treatment and service use differs by age, gender, ethnicity/race and education, *Social Psychiatry and Psychiatric Epidemiology*, 46: 45–57.

Goodspeed, R.B. and DeLucia, A.G. (1990) Stress reduction at the worksite: an evaluation of two methods, *American Journal of Health Promotion*, 4: 333–337.

Gordon, R. (ed) (1987) *An Operational Classification of Disease Prevention*. Rockville, MD: US Department of Health and Human Services.

Granot, D. and Mayseless, O. (2001) Attachment security and adjustment to school in middle childhood, *International Journal of Behavioral Development*, 25: 530–541.

Grantham-McGregor, S. (2007) Early child development in developing countries, *Lancet*, 369: 824.

Grantham-McGregor, S., Cheung, Y.B., Cueto, S., Glewwe, P., Richter, L. and Strupp, B. (2007) Developmental potential in the first 5 years for children in developing countries, *Lancet*, 369: 60–70.

Gray, J.A. (2002) Stigma in psychiatry, *Journal of the Royal Society of Medicine*, 95: 72–76.

Green, J. and Goldwyn, R. (2002) Annotation: attachment disorganisation and psychopathology: new findings in attachment research and their potential implications for developmental psychopathology in childhood, *Journal of Child Psychology and Psychiatry*, 43: 835–846.

Greenberg, M.T., Kusche, C.A., Cook, E.T. and Quamma, J.P. (1995) Promoting emotional competence in school-aged children: the effects of the PATHS curriculum, *Development and Psychology*, 7: 117–136.

Greenberg, M.T., Weissberg, R.P., O'Brien, M.U., Zins, J.E., Fredericks, L., Resnik, H. and Elias, M.J. (2003a) Enhancing school-based prevention and youth development through coordinated social, emotional, and academic learning, *American Psychologist*, 58: 466–474.

Greenberg, P.E., Kessler, R.C., Birnbaum, H.G., Leong, S.A., Lowe, S.W., Berglund, P.A. and Corey-Lisle, P.K. (2003b) The economic burden of depression in the United States: How did it change between 1990 and 2000?, *Journal of Clinical Psychiatry*, 64: 1465–1475.

Greenwald, A.G. and Nosek, B.A. (2009) Attitudinal dissociation: what does it mean?, in R.E. Petty, R.H. Fazio and P. Brinol (eds), *Attitudes: Insights from the New Implicit Measures* (pp. 65–82). Hillsdale, NJ: Erlbaum.

Greenwald, A.G., Poehlman, T.A., Uhlmann, E. and Banaji, M.R. (2009) Understanding and using the Implicit Association Test: III. Meta-analysis of predictive validity, *Journal of Personality and Social Psychology*, 97: 17–41.

Grienenberger, J., Kelly, K. and Slade, A. (2001) *Maternal Reflective Functioning and the Care-Giving Relationship: The Link between Mental States and Mother-Infant Affective Communication*. Paper presented at the Biennial Meeting of the Society for Research in Child Development, Minneapolis, MN.

Grossman, P., Niemann, L., Schmidt, S. and Walach, H. (2004) Mindfulness based stress reduction and health benefits: a meta-analysis, *Journal of Psychosomatic Research*, 57: 35–43.

Gulliver, A., Griffiths, K.M. and Christensen, H. (2010) Perceived barriers and facilitators to mental health help-seeking in young people: a systematic review, *BMC Psychiatry*, 10: 113.

Gyani, A., Shafran, R., Layard, R. and Clark, D.M. (2011) *Enhancing Recovery Rates in IAPT Services: Lessons from Analysis of the Year One Data*. London: National Health Service.

Haddon, W. Jr (1970) On the escape of tigers: an ecologic note, *American Journal of Public Health*, 60: 2229–2234.

Haddon, W. Jr (1980) Options for the prevention of motor vehicle crash injury, *Israel Journal of Medical Sciences*, 16: 45–65.

Haller, D.M., Sanci, L.A., Sawyer, S.M. and Patton, G.C. (2009) The identification of young people's emotional distress: a study in primary care, *British Journal of General Practice*, 59: e61–e70.

Hanlon, P. and Carlisle, S. (2009) Is modern culture bad for our well-being? *Global Health Promotion*, 16: 27–34.

Harris, E.C. and Barraclough, B. (1997) Suicide as an outcome for mental disorders. *British Journal of Psychiatry*, 170: 205–228.

Harris, R., Tobias, M., Jeffreys, M., Waldegrave, K., Karlsen, S. and Nazroo, J. (2005) *Maori Health and Inequalities in New Zealand: The Impact of Racism and Deprivation*. Wellington: Ministry of Health.

Harris, R., Tobias, M., Jeffreys, M., Waldegrave, K., Karlsen, S. and Nazroo, J. (2006) Racism and health: the relationship between experience of racial discrimination and health in New Zealand, *Social Science and Medicine*, 63: 1428–1441.

Harrison, P. (1993) *The Third Revolution: Population, Environment and a Sustainable World*. London: Penguin Books.

Hart, L.M., Jorm, A.F., Kanowski, J.G., Kelly, C.M. and Langlands, R.L. (2009) Mental health first aid for Indigenous Australians: using Delphi consensus studies to develop guidelines for culturally appropriate responses to mental health problems, *BMC Psychiatry*, 9: 47.

Hartmut, R. (1998) On defining the good life: liberal freedom and capitalist necessity, *Constellations*, 5: 201–214.

Harvey, S.B., Glozier, N., Henderson, M., Allaway, S., Litchfield, P., Holland-Elliott, K. and Hotopf, M. (2011) Depression and work performance: an ecological study using web-based screening, *Occupational Medicine*, 61: 209–211.

Haworth, J. and Hart, G. (2007) *Wellbeing: Individual, Community and Social Perspectives*. Basingstoke: Palgrave MacMillan.

Hayes, L., Smart, D., Toumbourou, J.W. and Sanson, A. (2004) *Parenting Influences on Adolescent Alcohol Use*. Melbourne: Australian Institute of Family Studies.

Hazan, C. and Shaver, P. (1987) Romantic love conceptualized as an attachment process, *Journal of Personality and Social Psychology*, 52: 511–524.

Health and Safety Executive (2009) *Stress Management Competency Indicator Tool*. London: Crown Copyright. Available at www.hse.gov.uk/stress/mcit.pdf (accessed 1 October 2012).

Hegerl, U., Mergl, R., Havers, I., Schmidtke, A., Lehfeld, H., Niklewski, G. and Althaus, D. (2010) Sustainable effects on suicidality were found for the Nuremberg alliance against depression, *European Archives of Psychiatry and Clinical Neuroscience*, 260: 401–406.

HelpAge International (2006) *Why Social Pensions are Needed Now*. London: HelpAge International.

Henderson, C. and Thornicroft, G. (2009) Stigma and discrimination in mental illness: Time to Change, *Lancet*, 373: 1930–1932.

Henderson, C., Liu, X., Diez Roux, A.V., Link, B.G. and Hasin, D. (2004) The effects of US state income inequality and alcohol policies on symptoms of depression and alcohol dependence, *Social Science and Medicine*, 58: 565–575.

Henderson, N. and Milstein, M. (2003) *Resiliency in Schools: Making it Happen for Students and Educators*. Thousand Oaks, CA: Corwin Press.

Hickie, I.B., Davenport, T.A. and Ricci, C.S. (2002) Screening for depression in general practice and related medical settings, *Medical Journal of Australia*, 177: 111–116.

Hinshaw, S.P. (2007) *The Mark of Shame: Stigma of Mental Illness and an Agenda for Change*. Oxford: Oxford University Press.

Hoddinott, J., Maluccio, J.A., Behrman, J.R., Flores, R. and Martorell, R. (2008) Effect of a nutrition intervention during early childhood on economic productivity in Guatemalan adults, *Lancet*, 371: 411–416.

Hogan, A., O'Loughlin, K., Miller, P.M. and Kendig, H. (2009) The health impact of a hearing disability on older people in Australia, *Journal of Aging and Health*, 21: 1098–1111.

Howe, D. (2010) *Attachment Across the Lifecourse: A Brief Introduction*. Basingstoke: Palgrave Macmillan.

Hu, Y., Stewart-Brown, S., Twigg, L. and Weich, S. (2007) Can the 12 item General Health Questionnaire be used to measure positive mental health?, *Psychological Medicine*, 37: 1005–1013.

Hubbert, M.K. (1945) Energy from fossil fuels, *Science*, 109: 103–109.

Huber, M., Knottnerus, J.A., Green, L., van der Horst, H., Jadad, A.R., Kromhout, D., Leonard, B., Lorig, K., Loureiro, M.I., van der Meer, J.W., Schnabel, P., Smith. R., van Weel, C. and Smid, H. (2011) How should we define health?, *British Medical Journal*, 343: d4163.

Hubley, J. and Copeman, J. (2008) *Practical Health Promotion*. Cambridge: Polity Press.

Humphrey, N., Kalambouka, A., Bolton, J., Lendrum, A., Wigelsworth, M., Lennie, C. and Farrell, P. (2008) *Primary Social and Emotional Aspects of Learning (SEAL): Evaluation of Small Group Work*. Manchester: School of Education, University of Manchester.

Huppert, F. (2005) Positive mental health in individuals and populations, in F. Huppert, N. Bayliss and B. Keverne (eds), *The Science of Wellbeing*. Oxford: Oxford University Press.

Hutchinson, E.D. (2011) *Dimensions of Human Behavior. The Changing Life Course*, 4th edn. Thousand Oaks, CA: Sage.

Insel, T.R. (2009) Translating scientific opportunity into public health impact: a strategic plan for research on mental illness, *Archives of General Psychiatry*, 66: 128–133.

Institute of Medicine (2002) *Reducing Suicide: A National Imperative*. Washington DC: The National Academies Press.

Intergovernmental Panel on Climate Change (2007) *Fourth Assessment Report*. New York: Cambridge University Press.

Jacobsen, N. and Greenley, D. (2001) What is recovery? A conceptual model and explication, *Psychiatric Services*, 52: 482–485.

Jacobvitz, D., Hazen, N.L. and Riggs, S. (1997) *Disorganized Mental Processes in Mothers, Frightened/Frightening Behavior in Caregivers, and Disoriented, Disorganized Behavior in Infancy*. Paper presented at the Biennial Meeting of the Society for Research in Child Development, Washington, DC.

Jahoda, M. (1958) *Current Concepts of Positive Mental Health*. New York: Basic Books.

James, O. (2007) *Affluenza: How to be Successful and Stay Sane*. London: Vermilion Books.

Jenkins, R. (2002) Addressing suicide as a public-health problem, *Lancet*, 359: 813–814.

Joa, I., Johannessen, J.O., Auestad, B., Friis, S., McGlashan, T., Melle, I., Opjordsmoen, S., Simonsen, E., Vaglum, P. and Larsen, T.K. (2008) The key to reducing duration of untreated first psychosis: information campaigns, *Schizophrenia Bulletin*, 34: 466–472.

Jorm, A.F. (2000) Mental health literacy. Public knowledge and beliefs about mental disorders, *British Journal of Psychiatry*, 177: 396–401.

Jorm, A.F. and Kitchener, B.A. (2011) Noting a landmark achievement: Mental health first aid training reaches 1% of Australian adults, *Australian and New Zealand Journal of Psychiatry*, 45: 808–813.

Jorm, A.F. and Wright, A. (2007) Beliefs of young people and their parents about the effectiveness of interventions for mental disorders, *Australian and New Zealand Journal of Psychiatry*, 41: 656–666.

Jorm, A.F., Angermeyer, M. and Katschnig, H. (2000a) Public knowledge and attitudes to mental disorders: a limiting factor in the optimal use of treatment services, in G. Andrews and A.S. Henderson (eds), *Unmet Need in Psychiatry*. Cambridge: Cambridge University Press.

Jorm, A.F., Christensen, H. and Griffiths, K.M. (2005c) The impact of beyondblue: the national depression initiative on the Australian public's recognition of depression and beliefs about treatments, *Australian and New Zealand Journal of Psychiatry*, 39: 248–254.

Jorm, A.F., Christensen, H. and Griffiths, K.M. (2006b) The public's ability to recognize mental disorders and their beliefs about treatment: changes in Australia over 8 years, *Australian and New Zealand Journal of Psychiatry*, 40: 36–41.

Jorm, A.F., Christensen, H. and Griffiths, K.M. (2006c) Changes in depression awareness and attitudes in Australia: the impact of beyondblue: the national depression initiative, *Australian and New Zealand Journal of Psychiatry*, 40: 42–46.

Jorm, A.F., Morgan, A.J. and Wright, A. (2008) Interventions that are helpful for depression and anxiety in young people: a comparison of clinicians' beliefs with those of youth and their parents, *Journal of Affective Disorders*, 111: 227–234.

Jorm, A.F., Kitchener, B.A., Fischer, J.A. and Cvetkovski, S. (2010a) Mental health first aid training by e-learning: a randomized controlled trial, *Australian and New Zealand Journal of Psychiatry*, 44: 1072–1081.

Jorm, A.F., Christensen, H., Griffiths, K.M. and Rodgers, B. (2002) Effectiveness of complementary and self-help treatments for depression, *Medical Journal of Australia*, 176: S84–S96.

Jorm, A.F., Kitchener, B.A., O'Kearney, R. and Dear, K.B. (2004) Mental health first aid training of the public in a rural area: a cluster randomized trial, *BMC Psychiatry*, 4: 33.

Jorm, A.F., Blewitt, K.A., Griffiths, K.M., Kitchener, B.A. and Parslow, R.A. (2005b) Mental health first aid responses of the public: results from an Australian national survey, *BMC Psychiatry*, 5: 9.

Jorm, A.F., Kitchener, B.A., Sawyer, M.G., Scales, H. and Cvetkovski, S. (2010b) Mental health first aid training for high school teachers: a cluster randomized trial, *BMC Psychiatry*, 10: 51.

Jorm, A.F., Kelly, C.M., Wright, A., Parslow, R.A., Harris, M.G. and McGorry, P.D. (2006a) Belief in dealing with depression alone: results from community surveys of adolescents and adults, *Journal of Affective Disorders*, 96: 59–65.

Jorm, A.F., Korten, A.E., Jacomb, P.A., Christensen, H., Rodgers, B. and Pollitt, P. (1997) Mental health literacy: a survey of the public's ability to recognise mental disorders and their beliefs about the effectiveness of treatment, *Medical Journal of Australia*, 166: 182–186.

Jorm, A.F., Medway, J., Christensen, H., Korten, A.E., Jacomb, P.A. and Rodgers, B. (2000b) Public beliefs about the helpfulness of interventions for depression: effects on actions taken when experiencing anxiety and depression symptoms, *Australian and New Zealand Journal of Psychiatry*, 34: 619–626.

Jorm, A.F., Nakane, Y., Christensen, H., Yoshioka, K., Griffiths, K.M. and Wata, Y. (2005a) Public beliefs about treatment and outcome of mental disorders: a comparison of Australia and Japan, *BMC Medicine*, 3: 12.

Kabat-Zim, J. (2003) Mindfulness-based interventions in context: Past, present and future, *Clinical Psychology Science and Practice*, 2: 44–56.

Kahn, R.S., Wise, P.H., Kennedy, B.P. and Kawachi, I. (2000) State income inequality, household income, and maternal mental and physical health: cross sectional national survey, *British Medical Journal*, 321: 1311–1315.

Kahneman, D. (1999) Objective happiness, in D. Kahnemann, E. Diener and N. Schwartz (eds), *Wellbeing: The Foundations of Hedonic Psychology*. New York: Russell Sage Foundation.

Kahneman, D., Krueger, A.B., Schkade, D.A., Schwarz, N. and Stone, A.A.I. (2004) A survey method for characterizing daily life experience: the day reconstruction method, *Science*, 306(5702): 1776–1780.

Kataoka, S.H., Zhang, L. and Wells, K.B. (2002) Unmet need for mental health care among U.S. children: variation by ethnicity and insurance status, *American Journal of Psychiatry*, 159: 1548–1555.

Katon, W. and Schulberg, H. (1992) Epidemiology of depression in primary care, *General Hospital Psychiatry*, 14: 237–247.

Katon, W., Von Korff, M., Lin, E., Walker, E., Simon, G.E., Bush, T., Robinson, P. and Russo, J. (1995) Collaborative management to achieve treatment guidelines: impact on depression in primary care, *Journal of the American Medical Association*, 273: 1026–1031.

Katon, W., Robinson, P., Von Korff, M., Lin, E., Bush, T., Ludman, E., Simon, G. and Walker, E. (1996) A multifaceted intervention to improve treatment of depression in primary care, *Archives of General Psychiatry*, 53: 924–32.

Katon, W., Von Korff, M., Lin, E., Simon, G., Walker, E., Unützer, J., Bush, T., Russo, J. and Ludman, E. (1999) Stepped collaborative care for primary care patients with persistent symptoms of depression: a randomized trial, *Archives of General Psychiatry*, 56: 1109–1115.

Kearns, A., Petticrew, M., Mason, P. and Whitley, E. (2008) *SHARP Survey Findings: Mental Health and Wellbeing Outcomes*. Edinburgh: Scottish Government Social Research.

Keitner, G.I., Ryan, C.E., Miller, I.W., Kohn, R., Bishop, D.S. and Epstein, N.B. (1995) Role of the family in recovery and major depression, *American Journal of Psychiatry*, 152: 1002–1008.

Kellam, S.G. and Langevin, D.J. (2003) A framework for understanding 'evidence' in prevention research and programs, *Prevention Science*, 4: 137–153.

Kelly, C.M., Jorm, A.F. and Rodgers, B. (2006) Adolescents' responses to peers with depression or conduct disorder, *Australian and New Zealand Journal of Psychiatry*, 40: 63–66.

Kelly, C.M., Jorm, A.F., Kitchener, B.A. and Langlands, R.L. (2008a) Development of mental health first aid guidelines for deliberate non-suicidal self-injury: a Delphi study, *BMC Psychiatry*, 8: 62.

Kelly, C.M., Jorm, A.F., Kitchener, B.A. and Langlands, R.L. (2008b) Development of mental health first aid guidelines for suicidal ideation and behaviour: a Delphi study, *BMC Psychiatry*, 8: 17.

Kelly, C.M., Jorm, A.F. and Kitchener, B.A. (2009) Development of mental health first aid guidelines for panic attacks: a Delphi study, *BMC Psychiatry*, 9: 49.

Kelly, C.M., Jorm, A.F. and Kitchener, B.A. (2010) Development of mental health first aid guidelines on how a member of the public can support a person affected by a traumatic event: a Delphi study, *BMC Psychiatry*, 10: 49.

Kelly, J.B. (2000) Children's adjustment in conflicted marriage and divorce: a decade review of research, *Journal of the American Academy of Child and Adolescent Psychiatry*, 39: 963–973.

Kennedy, H., Landor, M. and Todd, L. (2011) *Video-Interaction Guidance: A Relationship Based Intervention to Promote Attunement, Empathy and Wellbeing*. London: Jessica Kingsley Publisher.

Kennedy, R.F. (1968) University of Kansas Speech. Boston, MA: John F. Kennedy Presidential Library and Museum. Available at www.jfklibrary.org/Historical+Resources/Archives/Reference+Desk/Speeches/RFK/RFKSpeech68Mar18UKansas.htm (accessed 1 October 2012).

Kessing, L.V., Hansen, H.V., Demyttenaere, K. and Beck, P. (2005) Depressive and bipolar disorders: patients' attitudes and beliefs towards depression and antidepressants, *Psychological Medicine*, 35: 1205–1213.

Kessler, R. (2009) Identifying and screening for psychological and comorbid medical and psychological disorders in medical settings, *Journal of Clinical Psychology*, 65: 253–267.

Kessler, R.C. and Ustun, T.B. (eds) (2008) *The WHO World Mental Health Surveys: Global Perspectives on the Epidemiology of Mental Disorders*. New York: Cambridge University Press.

Kessler, R.C., Berglund, P., Demler, O., Jin, R., Koretz, D., Merikangas, K.R., Rush, A.J., Walters, E.E., Wang, P.S.; National Comorbidity Survey Replication (2003) The epidemiology of major depressive disorder: results from the National Comorbidity Survey Replication (NCS-R), *Journal of the American Medical Association*, 289: 3095–3105.

Kessler, R.C., Chiu, W.T., Demler, O., Merikangas, K.R. and Walters, E.E. (2005a) Prevalence, severity, and comorbidity of 12-month DSM-IV disorders in the National Comorbidity Survey Replication, *Archives of General Psychiatry*, 62: 617–627.

Kessler, R.C., Berglund, P., Demler, O., Jin, R., Merikangas, K.R. and Walters, E.E. (2005b) Lifetime prevalence and age-of-onset distributions of DSM-IV disorders in the National Comorbidity Survey Replication, *Archives of General Psychiatry*, 62: 593–602.

Kessler, R.C., Angermeyer, M., Anthony, J.C., De Graaf, R., Demytenaere, K., Gasquet, I., De Girolamo, G., Gluzman, S., Gureje, O., Haro, J.M., Kawakami, N., Karam, A., Levinson, D., Medina Mora, M.E., Oakley Browne, M.A., Posada-Villa, J., Stein, D.J., Adley Tsang, C.H., Aguilar-Gaxiola, S., Alonso, J., Lee, S., Heeringa, S., Pennell, B.E., Berglund, P., Gruber, M.J., Petukhova, M., Chatterji, S. and Ustün, T.B. (2007) Lifetime prevalence and age-of-onset distributions of mental disorders in the World Health Organization's World Mental Health Survey Initiative, *World Psychiatry*, 6: 168–176.

Kessler, R.C., Aguilar-Gaxiola, S., Alonso, J., Chatterji, S., Lee, S., Ormel, J., Ustün, T.B. and Wang, P.S. (2009) The global burden of mental disorders: an update from the WHO World Mental Health (WMH) surveys, *Epidemiologia e Psichiatria Sociale*, 18: 23–33.

Keyes, C.L.M. (2002) The mental health continuum: from languishing to flourishing in life, *Journal of Health and Social Research*, 43: 207–222.

Keyes, C.L.M. (2007) Promoting and protecting mental health as flourishing: a complementary strategy for improving national mental health, *American Psychologist*, 62: 95–108.

Keyes, C.L.M., Shmotkin, D. and Ryff, C.D. (2002) Optimizing wellbeing: the empirical encounter of two traditions, *Journal of Personality and Social Psychology*, 82: 1007–1022.

Killaspy, H., Bebbington, P., Blizard, B., Johnson, S., Nolan, F., Piling, S. and King, M. (2006) The REACT Study: randomised evaluation of assertive community treatment in North London, *British Medical Journal*, 332: 815–819.

King, M., Walker, C., Levy, G., Bottomley, C., Royston, P., Weich, S., Bellón-Saameño, J.A., Moreno, B., Svab, I., Rotar, D., Rifel, J., Maaroos, H.I., Aluoja, A., Kalda, R., Neeleman, J., Geerlings, M.I., Xavier, M., Carraça, I., Gonçalves-Pereira, M., Vicente, B., Saldivia, S., Melipillan, R., Torres-Gonzalez, F. and Nazareth, I. (2008) Development and validation of an international risk prediction algorithm for episodes of major depression in general practice attendees: the predictD study, *Archives of General Psychiatry*, 65: 1368–1376.

Kingston, A.H., Jorm, A.F., Kitchener, B.A., Hides, L., Kelly, C.M., Morgan, A.J., Hart, L.M. and Lubman, D.I. (2009) Helping someone with problem drinking: mental health first aid guidelines – a Delphi expert consensus study, *BMC Psychiatry*, 9: 79.

Kirsch, I. and Sapirstein, G. (1998) Listening to Prozac but hearing placebo: a meta-analysis of antidepressant medication, *Prevention and Treatment*, 1: 0002a.

Kirsch, I., Deacon, B.J., Huedo-Medina, T.B., Scoboria, A, Moore, T.J. and Johnson, J.B. (2008) Initial severity and antidepressant benefits: a meta-analysis of data submitted to the Food and Drug Administration, *PLoS Medicine*, 5/2: e45.

Kitchener, B.A. and Jorm, A.F. (2002) Mental health first aid training for the public: evaluation of effects on knowledge, attitudes and helping behavior, *BMC Psychiatry*, 2: 10.

Kitchener, B.A. and Jorm, A.F. (2004) Mental health first aid training in a workplace setting: a randomized controlled trial, *BMC Psychiatry*, 4: 23.

Kitchener, B.A. and Jorm, A.F. (2008) Mental health first aid: an international programme for early intervention, *Early Intervention in Psychiatry*, 2: 55–61.

Klein, M. and Grossman, S. (1971) Voting competence and mental illness, *American Journal of Psychiatry*, 127: 1562–1565.

Klem, A. and Connell, J. (2004) Relationships matter: linking teacher support to student engagement and achievement, *Journal of School Health*, 747: 262–273.

Knapp, M., Bauer, A., Perkins, M. and Snell, T. (2010) *Building Community Capacity: Making an Economic Case*. Personal Social Services Research Unit Discussion Paper 277229. Available at www.pssru.ac.uk/pdf/dp2772.pdf (accessed 21 August 2012).

Knapp, M., McDaid, D. and Parsonage, M. (2011) *Mental Health Promotion and Mental Illness Prevention: The Economic Case*. London: Department of Health.

Knifton, L. (2012) Understanding and addressing the stigma of mental illness with ethnic minority communities, *Health Sociology Review*, 21: 287–298.

Knifton, L., Gervais, M., Newbigging, K., Mirza, N., Quinn, N., Wilson, N. and Hunkins-Hutchison, E. (2010) Community conversation: addressing mental health stigma with ethnic minority communities, *Social Psychiatry and Psychiatric Epidemiology*, 45: 497–504.

Knox, K.L., Conwell, Y. and Caine, E.D. (2004) If suicide is a public health problem, what are we doing to prevent it?, *American Journal of Public Health*, 94: 37–45.

Kondo, N., Sembajwe, G., Kawachi, I., van Dam, R.M., Subramanian, S.V. and Yamagata, Z. (2009) Income inequality, mortality and self-rated health: a meta-analysis of multilevel studies with 60 million subjects, *British Medical Journal*, 339: b4471.

Koponen, H.J., Viilo, K., Hakko, H., Timonen, M., Meyer-Rochow, V.B., Sarkioja, T. and Räsänen, P. (2007) Rates and previous disease history in old age suicide, *International Journal of Geriatric Psychiatry*, 24: 916–920.

Kovess-Masfety, V., Saragoussi, D., Sevilla-Dedieu, C., Gilbert, F., Suchocka, A., Arveiller, N., Gasquet, I., Younes, N. and Hardy-Bayle, M.C. (2007) What makes people decide who to turn to when faced with a mental health problem? Results from a French survey, *BMC Public Health*, 7: 188.

Kreitman, N. (1976) The coal gas story: United Kingdom suicide rates, 1960–71, *British Journal of Preventive and Social Medicine*, 30: 86–93.

Kretzman, J. and McKnight, J. (1993) *Building Communities from the Inside Out: A Path Toward Finding and Mobilizing a Community's Assets*. Evanston, IL: ACTA Publications.

Lae, A. and Crano, W.D. (2009) Monitoring matters: a meta-analytic review reveals the reliable linkage of parental monitoring with adolescent marijuana use, *Perspectives on Psychological Science*, 4: 578–586.

Lane, R.E. (2000) *The Loss of Happiness in Market Democracies*. London: Yale University Press.

Lang, G., Resch, K., Hofer, K., Braddick, F. and Gabilondo, A. (2010) *Background Document for the Thematic Conference on Mental Health and Well-being among Older People*. Luxembourg: European Communities.

Langlands, R.L., Jorm, A.F., Kelly, C.M. and Kitchener, B.A. (2008) First aid for depression: a Delphi consensus study with consumers, carers and clinicians, *Journal of Affective Disorders*, 105: 157–165.

Lapsley, H., Nikora, L. and Black, R. (2002) *Kia Mauri Tau: Narratives of Recovery from Disabling Mental Health Problems*. Wellington: Mental Health Commission.

Larkin, G.L., Hamann, C.J., Monico, E.P., Degutis, L., Schuur, J., Kantor, W. and Graffeo, C.S. (2007) Knowledge translation at the macro level: legal and ethical considerations, *Academic Emergency Medicine*, 14: 1042–1046.

Lasch, C. (1979) *The Culture of Narcissism: American Life in an Age of Diminishing Expectations*. London: WW Norton.

Lauber, C., Nordt, C., Falcato, L. and Rossler, W. (2001) Lay recommendations on how to treat mental disorders, *Social Psychiatry and Psychiatric Epidemiology*, 36: 553–556.

Lawrence, D. and Kisely, S. (2010) Review: inequalities in healthcare provision for people with severe mental illness, *Journal of Psychopharmacology*, 24: 61–68.

Layard, R. (2005) *Happiness: Lessons from a New Science*. London: Allen Lane.

Leaf, P.J., Schultz, D., Kiser, L.J. and Pruitt, D.B. (2003) School mental health in systems of care, in M.D. Weist, S.W. Evans and N.A. Lever (eds), *Handbook of School Mental Health Programs: Advancing Practice and Research* (pp. 239–256). New York: Springer.

Lecce, S. (2008) *Attachment and Subjective Well-Being: the Mediating Role of Emotional Processing and Regulation*. Toronto: University of Toronto.

Lee, S., Chiu, M.Y., Tsang, A., Chui, H. and Kleinman, A. (2006) Stigmatizing experience and structural discrimination associated with the treatment of schizophrenia in Hong Kong, *Social Science and Medicine*, 62: 1685–1696.

Leinonen, T., Pietilainen, O., Laaksonen, M., Rahkonen, O., Lahelma, E. and Martikainen, P. (2011) Occupational social class and disability retirement among municipal employees – the contribution of health behaviors and working conditions, *Scandinavian Journal of Work Environment and Health*, 37: 464–472.

Lieberman, A.F. and Amaya-Jackson, L. (2005) Reciprocal influences of attachment and trauma: using a dual lens in the assessment and treatment of infants, toddler and preschools, in E.B. Foa, T.M. Kean, M.J. Friedman and J.A. Cohen (eds), *Effective Treatment for PTSD: Predictive Guidelines from the International Society for Traumatic Stress Studies*, 2nd edn. New York: Guilford Press.

Lima, M.S. and Moncrief, J. (2003) Drugs versus placebo for dysthymia, in *The Cochrane Library, Issue 2*. Chichester: John Wiley and Sons.

Lindstrom, B. and Eriksson, M. (2005) Salutogenesis, *Journal of Epidemiology and Community Health*, 59: 440–442.

Link, B.G. and Phelan, J.C. (2001) Conceptualizing stigma, *Annual Review of Sociology*, 27: 363–385.

Link, B.G., Mirotznik, J. and Cullen, F.T. (1991) The effectiveness of stigma coping orientations: Can negative consequences of mental illness labeling be avoided?, *Journal of Health and Social Behavior*, 32: 302–320.

Link, B.G., Yang, L.H., Phelan. J.C. and Collins, P.Y. (2004) Measuring mental illness stigma, *Schizophrenia Bulletin*, 30: 511–541.

Linley, A. and Joseph, S. (2004) *Positive Psychology and Practice*. Hoboken, NJ: John Wiley and Sons.

Lloyd-Evans, B., Crosby, M., Stockton, S., Piling, S., Hobbs, L., Hinton, M. and Johnson, S. (2011) Initiatives to reduce the duration of untreated psychosis: a systematic review, *British Journal of Psychiatry*, 198: 256–263.

Local Government Improvement and Development (LGID) (2010) *The Role of Local Government in Promoting Wellbeing*. London: LGID. Available: www.idea.gov.uk/idk/aio/23693073 (accessed 21 August 2012).

Ludwig, D.S. and Kabat-Zim, J. (2008) Mindfulness in medicine, *Journal of the American Medical Association*, 300: 1350–1352.

Lund, C., Breen, A., Flisher, A.J., Kakuma, R., Corrigall, J., Joska, J.A., Swartz, l. and Patel, V. (2010) Poverty and common mental disorders in low and middle income countries: a systematic review, *Social Science and Medicine*, 71: 517–528.

Lund, C., de Silva, M., Plagerson, S., Cooper, S., Chisholm, D., Das, J., Knapp, M. and Patel, V. (2011) Poverty and mental disorders: breaking the cycle in low-income and middle-income countries, *Lancet*, 378: 1502–1514.

Lundberg, U. and Cooper, C.L. (2011) *The Science of Occupational Health*. Oxford: Wiley-Blackwell.

Lury, C. (2003) *Consumer Culture*. Cambridge: Polity Press.

Lykken, D. (1999) *Happiness: What Studies on Twins show us about Nature, Nurture, and the Happiness Set-Point*. New York: Golden Books.

Lyons-Ruth, K., Yellin, C., Melnick, S. and Atwood, G. (2005) Expanding the concept of unresolved mental states: hostile/helpless states of mind on the Adult Attachment Interview are associated with disrupted mother-infant communication and infant disorganization, *Development and Psychopathology*, 17: 1–23.

Lyubomirsky, S. (2010) *The How of Happiness: A Practical Approach to Getting the Life You Want*. London: Piatkus.

Lyubomirsky, S. (2011) Hedonic adaptation to positive and negative experiences, in S. Folkman (ed.), *Oxford Handbook of Stress, Health, and Coping*. New York: Oxford University Press.

McCrone, P., Craig, T.K., Power, P. and Garety, P. (2010) Cost-effectiveness of an early intervention service for people with psychosis, *British Journal of Psychiatry*, 196: 377–382.

McDaid, D. (2008) *Mental Health in Workplace Settings*. Luxembourg: European Communities.

McDaid, D. (2011) *Background Document for the Thematic Conference on Promotion of Mental Health and Well-being in Workplaces*. Luxembourg: European Communities.

McDaid, D., Zechmeister, I., Kilian, R., Medeiros, H., Knapp, M., Kennelly, B. and the MHEEN Group (2007) *Making the Economic Case for the Promotion of Mental Well-being and the Prevention of Mental Health Problems*. London: London School of Economics and Political Science.

McGorry, P., Nordentoft, M. and Simonsen, E. (eds) (2005) Introduction to 'Early psychosis: a bridge to the future', *British Journal of Psychiatry*, 187 (Suppl 48): s1–s3.

McGorry, P., Hickie, I.B., Yung, A., Pantelis, C. and Jackson, H.J. (2006) Clinical staging of psychiatric disorders: a heuristic framework for choosing earlier, safer and more effective interventions, *Australian and New Zealand Journal of Psychiatry*, 40: 616–622.

McKee, S. and the Older Age Working Group (2010) *The Forgotten Age: Understanding Poverty and Social Exclusion Later in Life*. London: The Centre for Social Justice.

Mackinnon, A., Griffiths, K.M. and Christensen, H. (2008) Comparative randomised trial of online cognitive-behavioural therapy and an information website for depression: 12-month outcomes, *British Journal of Psychiatry*, 192: 130–134.

McMichael, A.J., Woodruff, R.E. and Hales, S. (2006) Climate change and human health: present and future risks, *Lancet*, 367: 859–869.

McNeill, A. (2001) *Smoking and Mental Health: A Review of the Literature*. London: SmokeFree.

MacQueen, K. and Cates, W. (2005) The multiple layers of prevention science research, *American Journal of Preventive Medicine*, 28: 491–495.

Madigan, M., Bakermans-Kranenburg, M., van Ijzendoorn, G., Moran, D.R., Pederson, D.R. and Benoit, D. (2006) Unresolved states of mind, anomalous parental behaviour and disorganized attachment: a review and meta-analysis of a transmission gap, *Attachment and Human Behavior*, 8: 89–111.

Magill-Evans, J., Harrison, M.J., Rempel. G. and Slater, L. (2006) Interventions with fathers of young children: systematic literature review, *Journal of Advanced Nursing*, 55: 248–264.

Magliano, L., Fiorillo, A., De Rosa, C., Malangone, C. and Maj, M. (2004) Beliefs about schizophrenia in Italy: a comparative nationwide survey of the general public, mental health professionals, and patients' relatives, *Canadian Journal of Psychiatry*, 49: 322–330.

Maheswaran, H., Powell, J., Weich, S. and Stewart-Brown, S. (in press) Establishing the responsiveness of the Warwick-Edinburgh Mental Well-being Scale (WEMWEBS): Group and individual level analysis, *Biomed Central Health and Quality of Life Outcomes*.

Main, M. and Hesse, E. (1990) Parents' unresolved traumatic experiences are related to infant disorganised attachment status: is frightening and/or frightened parental behaviour the linking mechanism?, in M. Greenberg, D. Cicchetti and E.M. Cummings (eds), *Attachment in the Preschool Years: Theory, Research and Intervention*. Chicago, IL: University of Chicago Press.

Main, M. and Solomon, J. (1986) Discovery of an insecure disorganized/disoriented attachment pattern: procedures, findings and implications for classification of behaviour, in M.W. Yogman and T.B. Brazelton (eds), *Affective Development in Infancy*. Norwood, NJ: Ablex.

Major, B. and O'Brien, L.T. (2005) The social psychology of stigma, *Annual Review of Psychology*, 56: 393–421.

Mann, J.J., Apter, A., Bertolote, J., Beautrais, A., Currier, D., Haas, A., Hegerl, U., Lonnqvist, J., Malone, K., Marusic, A., Mehlum, L., Patton, G., Phillips, M., Rutz, W., Rihmer, Z., Schmidtke, A., Shaffer, D., Silverman, M., Takahashi, Y., Varnik, A., Wasserman, D., Yip, P. and Hendin, H. (2005) Suicide prevention strategies: a systematic review, *Journal of the American Medical Association*, 294: 2064–2074.

Marks, N. and Shah, H. (2005) A wellbeing manifesto for a flourishing society, In F. Huppert, N. Baylis and B. Keverne (eds), *The New Science of Wellbeing*. Oxford: Oxford University Press.

Marmot, M. (2004) *The Status Syndrome: How Social Standing Affects our Health and Longevity*. New York: Times Books.

Marmot, M. (2010) *Fair Society, Healthy Lives: Strategic Review of Health Inequalities in England Post-2010. The Marmot Review*. London: The Marmot Review.

Marmot, M. and Wilkinson, R. (eds) (2006) *Social Determinants of Health*. Oxford: Oxford University Press.

Marsden, G., Cattan, M., Jopson, A. and Woodward, C. (2010) Do transport planning tools reflect the needs of the older traveller?, *Quality in Ageing and Older Adults*, 11: 16–24.

Marshall, M., Lewis, S., Lockwood, A., Drake, R., Jones, P. and Croudace, T. (2005) Association between duration of untreated psychosis and outcome in cohorts of first-episode patients: a systematic review, *Archives of General Psychiatry*, 62: 975–983.

Marwaha, S. and Johnson, S. (2004) Schizophrenia and employment, *Social Psychiatry and Psychiatric Epidemiology*, 39: 337–349.

Maxwell, M. (2005) General practitioners' and women's experiences of depression and its management in primary care: the moral dilemma of care, *Chronic Illness*, 1: 61–71.

Meins, E., Fernyhough, C., Fradley, E. and Tuckey, M. (2001) Rethinking maternal sensitivity: mothers' comments on infants' mental processes predict security of attachment at 12 months, *Journal of Child Psychology and Psychiatry*, 42: 637–648.

Mental Health Advocacy Coalition (2008) *Destination: Recovery: Te Ūnga ki Uta: Te Oranga*. Auckland: Mental Health Foundation of New Zealand.

Mental Health Commission (2004) *Our Lives in 2014: A Recovery Vision from People with Experience of Mental Illness*. Wellington: Mental Health Commission.

Merritt, R.K., Price, J.R., Mollison, J. and Geddes, J.R. (2007) A cluster randomized controlled trial to assess the effectiveness of an intervention to educate students about depression, *Psychological Medicine*, 37: 363–372.

Merz, E.M. and Consedine, N.S. (2009) The association of family support and wellbeing in later life depends on adult attachment style, *Attachment and Human Development*, 11: 203–221.

Mills, C., Mulloy, M. and Weist, M. (2010) Realizing the possibilities of school mental health across the public health continuum, in N. Cohen and S. Galea (eds), *Population Mental Health: Evidence, Policy, and Public Health Practice*. New York: Routledge.

Minkler, M. and Wallerstein, N. (2005) Improving health through community organisation and community building: a health education perspective, in M. Minkler (ed), *Community Organising and Community Building for Health*. New Brunswick, NJ: Rutgers University Press.

Mishara, B. and Ystgaard, M. (2006) Effectiveness of a mental health promotion program to improve coping skills in young children: Zippy's Friends, *Early Childhood Research Quarterly*, 21: 110–123.

Moessner, R., Mikova, O., Koutsilieri, E., Saoud, M., Ehlis, A.C., Müller, N., Fallgatter, A.J. and Riederer, P. (2007) Consensus paper of the WFSBP Task Force on Biological Markers: Biological Markers in Depression, *The World Journal of Biological Psychiatry*, 8: 141–174.

Moffatt, S. (2009) Work, retirement and money, in M. Cattan (ed), *Mental Health and Well-being in Later Life* (pp. 64–83). Maidenhead: Open University Press/McGraw-Hill.

Moffatt, S. and Scambler, S. (2008) Can welfare-rights advice targeted at older people reduce social exclusion?, *Ageing and Society*, 28: 875–899.

Mojtabai, R. (2007) Americans' attitudes toward mental health treatment seeking: 1990–2003, *Psychiatric Services*, 58: 642–651.

Mojtabai, R. (2009) Americans' attitudes toward psychiatric medications: 1998–2006, *Psychiatric Services*, 60: 1015–1023.

Moore, T.H., Zammit, S., Lingford-Hughes, A., Barnes, T.R., Jones, P.B., Burke M. and Lewis, G. (2007) Cannabis use and risk of psychotic or affective mental health outcomes: a systematic review, *Lancet*, 370: 319–328.

Morgan, D., Grant, K.A., Gage, H.D., Mach, R.H., Kaplan, J.R., Prioleau, O., Nader, S.H., Buchheimer, N., Ehrenkaufer, R.L. and Nader, M.A. (2002) Social dominance in monkeys: dopamine D2 receptors and cocaine self-administration, *Nature Neuroscience*, 5: 169–174.

Moss, E., Dubois-Comtois, K., Cyr, C., Tarabulsy, G.M., St-Laurent, D. and Bernier, A. (2011) Efficacy of a home-visiting intervention aimed at improving maternal sensitivity, child attachment, and behavioral outcomes for maltreated children: a randomized control trial, *Development and Psychopathology*, 23: 195–210.

Mrazek, P. and Haggerty, R. (eds) (1994) *Reducing Risks for Mental Disorders: Frontiers for Preventive Intervention Research*. Washington DC: Institute of Medicine, National Academy Press.

Mrazek. P.J. and Hosman, C.M. (eds) (2002) *Toward a Strategy for Worldwide Action to Promote Mental Health and Prevent Mental and Behavioral Disorders*. Alexandria, VA: World Federation for Mental Health.

Mufson, L.H., Dorta, K.P., Olfson, M., Weissman, M.M. and Hoagwood, K. (2004) Effectiveness research: transporting Interpersonal Psychotherapy for Depressed Adolescents (IPT-A) from the lab to school-based health clinics, *Clinical Child and Family Psychology Review*, 7: 251–261.

Mulloy, M. (2011) School-based resilience: how an urban public high school reduced students' exposure to risk and nurtured their social-emotional development and academic success, *Advances in School Mental Health Promotion*, 4: 4–22.

Munoz, R.F. (2010) Using evidence-based internet interventions to reduce health disparities worldwide, *Journal of Medical Internet Research*, 12: e60.

Murray, C.J. and Lopez, A.D. (1997) Alternative projections of mortality and disability by cause 1990–2020: Global Burden of Disease Study, *Lancet*, 349: 1498–1504.

Murray, L. and Andrews, L. (2005) *The Social Baby: Understanding Babies' Communications from Birth*. Richmond: CP Publishing.

Nash, M. (2005) Physical care skills: a training needs analysis of inpatient and community mental health nurses, *Mental Health Practice*, 9: 20–23.

Nash, M. (2011) Improving mental health service users' physical health through medication monitoring: a literature review, *Journal of Nursing Management*, 19: 360–365.

Nasrallah, H.A., Meyer, J.M., Goff, D.C., McEvoy, J.P., Davis, S.M., Stroup, T.S. and Lieberman, J.A. (2006) Low rates of treatment for hypertension, dyslipidaemia and diabetes in schizophrenia: data from the CATIE schizophrenia trial sample at baseline, *Schizophrenia Research*, 86: 15–22.

National Assembly on School-Based Health Care (2006) *School-Based Health Centers National Census School Year 2004–2005*. Washington: NASBHC.

National Institute for Health and Clinical Excellence (2006) *Depression and Anxiety – Computerised Cognitive Behaviour Therapy (CCBT)*. London: NICE.

National Institute for Health and Clinical Excellence (2008a) *Community Engagement to Improve Health*. London: NICE.

National Institute for Health and Clinical Excellence (2008b) *Occupational Therapy Interventions and Physical Activity Interventions to Promote the Mental Wellbeing of Older People in Primary Care and Residential Care*. London: NICE.

National Institute for Health and Clinical Excellence (2009a) *Depression in Adults*. CG90. London: NICE.

National Institute for Health and Clinical Excellence (2009b) *Depression with a Chronic Physical Health Problem*. CG91. London: NICE.

National Institute for Health and Clinical Excellence (2009c) *Promoting Wellbeing at Work – Public Health Guidance PH22*. London: NICE.

Nelson, T.D. (2009) *Handbook of Prejudice, Stereotyping and Discrimination*. New York: Psychology Press.

Nesse, R.N. (2005) Natural selection and the elusiveness of happiness, in F. Huppert, N. Baylis and B. Keverne (eds), *The New Science of Wellbeing*. Oxford: Oxford University Press.

New Economics Foundation (2004) *A Well-being Manifesto for a Flourishing Society*. London: New Economics Foundation.

New Economics Foundation (2008) *Measuring Well-being in Policy: Issues and Applictions*. London: New Economics Foundation.

New Economics Foundation (2009) *National Accounts of Wellbeing*. London: nef.

New Freedom Commission on Mental Health (2003) *Achieving the Promise: Transforming Mental Health Care in America (SMA-03–3832)*. Rockville, MD: Department of Health and Human Services.

NHS Ayrshire and Arran (2005) *Help Yourself to Better Health*. Scotland: Scottish Government.

NHS Clinical Knowledge Summaries (2011) *Depression*. Available at www.cks.nhs.uk/depression/ (accessed 24 August 2012).

NHS Information Centre for Health and Social Care (2009) *Adult Psychiatric Morbidity in England, 2007: Results of a Household Survey*. Leeds: NHS. Available at www.ic.nhs.uk/statistics-and-data-collections/mental-health/mental-health-surveys/adult-psychiatric-morbidity-in-england-2007-results-of-a-household-survey (accessed 30 September 2012).

Nock, M.K., Borges, G., Bromet, E.J., Alonso, J., Angermeyer, M., Beautrais, A., Bruffaerts, R., Chiu, W.T., de Girolamo, G., Gluzman, S., de Graaf, R., Gureje, O., Haro, J.M., Huang, Y., Karam, E., Kessler, R.C., Lepine, J.P., Levinson, D., Medina-Mora, M.E., Ono, Y., Posada-Villa, J. and Williams, D. (2008a) Cross-national prevalence and risk factors for suicidal ideation, plans and attempts, *British Journal of Psychiatry*, 192: 98–105.

Nock, M.K., Borges, G., Bromet, E.J., Cha, C.B., Kessler, R.C. and Lee, S. (2008b) Suicide and suicidal behavior, *Epidemiologic Reviews*, 30: 133–154.

Nosek, B.A. (2007) Implicit-explicit relations, *Current Directions in Psychological Science*, 16: 65–69.

O'Connell, M.E., Boat, T. and Warner, K.E. (eds) (2009) *Preventing Mental, Emotional and Behavioral Disorders Among Young People: Progress and Possibilities*. Washington DC: National Academies Press.

O'Hagan, M. (1994) *Stopovers on my Way Home from Mars: A Journey into the Psychiatric Survivor Movement in the USA, Britain and the Netherlands*. Available at www.maryohagan.com/publications (accessed 24 August 2012).

O'Hagan, M. (2001) *Recovery Competencies for New Zealand Mental Health Workers*. Wellington: Mental Health Commission.

O'Hagan, M. (2006) Guest editorial, *MindNet, Issue 4*. Auckland: Mental Health Foundation.

O'Connor, E.A., Whitlock, E.P., Beil, T.L. and Gaynes, B.N. (2009) Screening for depression in adult patients in primary care settings: a systematic evidence review, *Annals of Internal Medicine*, 151: 793–803.

Office for National Statistics (2000) *Psychiatric Morbidity among Adults living in Private Households* (p. 93). London: ONS.

Office for National Statistics (2001) *Psychiatric Morbidity among Adults Living in Private Households, 2000*. London: TSO.

Office for National Statistic (2011a) *Measuring National Well-Being: National Statistician's Reflections on the National Debate on Measuring National Well-Being*. London: ONS.

Office for National Statistics (2011b) *Older People's Day 2011*. London: ONS.

Office of the Deputy Prime Minister (2004) *Mental Health and Social Exclusion*. London: Social Exclusion Unit.

Onken, S., Dumont, J., Ridgway, P., Dornan, D. and Ralph, R. (2002) *Mental Health Recovery: What Helps and What Hinders?* Alexandria, VA: National Technical Assistance Center for State Mental Health Planning.

Organisation for Economic and Co-operative Development (2011a) *Better Life Index*. Paris: OECD. Available at www.oecdbetterlifeindex.org (accessed 22 August 2012).

Organisation for Economic Co-operation and Development (2011b) *Sick on the Job? Myths and Realities about Mental Health and Work*. Paris: Organisation for Economic Co-operation and Development (OECD) Publishing.

Oxford Economics (2007) *Mental Health and the UK Economy*. Oxford: Oxford Economics.

Palmer, G., North, J. and Kenway, P. (2003) *Monitoring Poverty and Social Exclusion*. York: Joseph Rowntree Foundation.

Palmer, S. and Dryden, W. (1994) Stress management: approaches and interventions, *British Journal of Guidance and Counselling*, 22: 5–11.

Parry-Jones, S. (2006) *Neighbourhood Accessibility, Social Networks and Mental Wellbeing: A Literature Review*. London: ARUP.

Parsonage, M. (2007) *The Impact of Mental Health on Business and Industry – An Economic Analysis*. London: Sainsbury Centre for Mental Health.

Patel, V. and Prince, M. (2010) Global mental health: a new global health field comes of age, *Journal of the American Medical Association*, 303: 1976–1977.

Patel, V., Lund, C., Hatherill, S., Plagerson, S., Corrigall, J., Funk, M. and Flisher, A.J. (2010) Mental disorders: equity and social determinants, in E. Blas and A.S. Kurup (eds), *Equity, Social Determinants and Public Health Programmes*. Geneva: WHO.

Paternite, C.E. and Chiara-Johnston, T. (2005) Rationale and strategies for the central involvement of educators in effective school-based mental health programs, *Journal of Youth and Adolescence*, 34: 41–49.

Pawson, R. and Tilley, N. (1997) *Realistic Evaluation*. London: Sage.

Pearse, I.H. and Williamson, G.S. (1938/1982) *Biologists in Search of Material – An Interim Report on the Work of the Pioneer Health Centre Peckham*. Edinburgh: Scottish Academic Press.

Perlis, T.E., Des Jarlais, D.C., Friedman, S.R., Arasteh, K. and Turner, C.F. (2004) Audio-computerized self-interviewing versus face-to-face interviewing for research data collection at drug abuse treatment programs, *Addiction*, 99: 885–896.

Pescosolido, B.A., Jensen, P.S., Martin, J.K., Perry, B.L., Olafsdottir, S. and Fettes, D. (2008) Public knowledge and assessment of child mental health problems: findings from the National Stigma Study-Children, *Journal of the American Academy of Child and Adolescent Psychiatry*, 47: 339–349.

Pescosolido, B.A., Martin, J.K., Long, J.S., Medina, T.R., Phelan, J.C. and Link, B.G. (2010) 'A disease like any other'? A decade of change in public reactions to schizophrenia, depression, and alcohol dependence, *American Journal of Psychiatry*, 167: 1321–1330.

Petersen, I. (2010) At the heart of development: an introduction to mental health promotion and the prevention of mental disorders in scarce-resource contexts, in I. Petersen, A. Bhana, A.J. Flisher, L. Swartz and L. Richter (eds), *Promoting Mental Health in Scarce-Resource Contexts. Emerging Evidence and Practice*. Cape Town: HSRC Press.

Petersen, I., Bhana, A., Flisher, A.J., Swartz, L. and Richter, L. (eds) (2010) *Promoting Mental Health in Scarce-Resource Contexts. Emerging Evidence and Practice*. Cape Town: HSRC Press.

Pettigrew, T.F. and Tropp, L.R. (2006) A meta-analytic test of intergroup contact theory, *Journal of Personality and Social Psychology*, 90: 751–783.

Phelan, J.C., Yang, L.H. and Cruz-Rojas, R. (2006) Effects of attributing serious mental illnesses to genetic causes on orientations to treatment, *Psychiatric Services*, 57: 382–387.

Phelan, M., Stradins, L. and Morrison, S. (2001) Physical health of people with severe mental illness, *British Medical Journal*, 322: 443–444.

Phillips, M.R., Li, X. and Zhang, Y. (2002) Suicide rates in China, 1995–99, *Lancet*, 359: 835–840.

Phillips, S., Brent, J., Kulig, K., Heiligenstein, J. and Birkett, M. (1997) Fluoxetine versus tricyclic antidepressants: a prospective multicenter study of antidepressant drug overdoses. The Antidepressant Study Group, *Journal of Emergency Medicine*, 15: 439–445.

Pignone, M.P., Gaynes, B.N., Rushton, J.L., Burchell, C.M., Orleans, C.T., Mulrow, C.D. and Lohr, K.N. (2002) Screening for depression in adults: a summary of the evidence for the U.S. Preventive Services Task Force, *Annals of Internal Medicine*, 136: 765–776.

Pinder, R., Kessel, A., Green, J. and Grundy, C. (2009) Exploring perceptions of health and the environment: a qualitative study of Thames Chase Community Forrest, *Health and Place*, 15: 349–356.

Pinfold, V., Toulmin, H., Thornicroft, G., Huxley, P., Farmer, P. and Graham, T. (2003) Reducing psychiatric stigma and discrimination: evaluation of educational interventions in UK secondary schools, *British Journal of Psychiatry*, 182: 342–346.

Pinfold, V., Byrne, P. and Toulmin, H. (2005) Challenging stigma and discrimination in communities: a focus group study identifying UK mental health service users' main campaign priorities, *International Journal of Social Psychiatry*, 51: 128–138.

Pinto-Foltz, M.D., Logsdon, M.C. and Myers, J.A. (2011) Feasibility, acceptability, and initial efficacy of a knowledge-contact program to reduce mental illness stigma and improve mental health literacy in adolescents, *Social Science and Medicine*, 72: 2011–2019.

Popay, J. (2010) Community engagement for health improvement: questions of definition, outcomes and evaluation, in A. Morgan, R. Barker, M. Davies and E. Ziglio (eds), *Health Assets in a Global Context: Theory, Methods, Action*. New York: Springer.

Popple, K. (1995) *Analysing Community Work: Its Theory and Practice*. Buckingham: Open University Press.

Porter, R. (2002) *Madness: A Brief History*. Oxford: Oxford University Press.

Priest, R.G., Vize, C., Roberts, A., Roberts, M. and Tylee, A. (1996) Lay people's attitudes to treatment of depression: results of opinion poll for Defeat Depression Campaign just before its launch, *British Medical Journal*, 313: 858–859.

Prince, M., Livingston, G. and Katona, C. (2007a) Mental health care for the elderly in low-income countries: a health systems approach, *World Psychiatry*, 6: 5–13.

Prince, M., Patel, V., Saxena, S., Maj, M., Maselko, J., Phillips, M.R. and Rahman, A. (2007b) No health without mental health, *Lancet*, 370: 859–877.

Prince, M.J. (2010) Older people, in I. Petersen, A. Petersen, A. Bhana, A.J. Flisher, L. Swartz and L. Richter (eds), *Promoting Mental Health in Scarce-Resource Contexts. Emerging Evidence and Practice*. Cape Town: HSRC Press.

Puckering, C., Rogers, J., Mills, M., Cox, A.D. and Mattsson-Graf, M. (1994) Process and evaluation of a group intervention for mothers with parenting difficulties, *Child Abuse Review*, 3: 299–310.

Putnam, R.D. (2000) *Bowling Alone: The Collapse and Revival of American Community*. New York: Simon and Schuster.

Pyne, J.M., Rost, K.M., Farahati, F., Tripathi, S.P., Smith, J., Williams, D.K., Fortney, J. and Coyne, J.C. (2005) One size fits some: the impact of patient treatment attitudes on the cost-effectiveness of a depression primary-care intervention, *Psychological Medicine*, 35: 839–854.

Quinn, N. (2010) The role of community development in tackling mental health inequalities, in I. Goldie (ed.), *Public Mental Health Today: A Handbook*. Brighton: Pavillion Publishing.

Quinn, N. and Knifton, L. (2012) Positive Mental Attitudes: how community development principles have shaped a 10-year mental health inequalities programme in the UK, *Community Development Journal*, 47: 588–603.

Quinn, N., Shulman, A., Knifton, L. and Byrne, P. (2011a) The impact of a national mental health arts and film festival on stigma and recovery, *Acta Psychiatrica Scandinavica*, 123: 71–81.

Quinn, N., Knifton, L. and Donald, J. (2011b) The role of personal narratives in addressing stigma, in R. Taylor, F. McNeill and M. Hill (eds) *Early Professional Development for Social Workers*. Birmingham: Venture Press.

Raeburn, J. (2008). *Aotearoa New Zealand: Charter for Mental Health Promotion*. Unpublished document.

Rahman, A., Mubbashar, M.H., Gater, R. and Goldberg, D. (1998) Randomised trial of impact of school mental-health programme in rural Rawalpindi, Pakistan, *Lancet*, 352: 1022–1025.

Rajala, M. (2001) European developments in health promotion, *Promotion and Education*, Supplement, 5–6.

Ransome, P. (2005) *Work, Consumption and Culture: Affluence and Social Change in the 21st Century*. London: Sage.

Raphael, D. (2000) The question of evidence in health promotion, *Health Promotion International*, 15: 355–367.

Read, J., Mosher, L. and Bentall, R. (2004) *Models of Madness: Psychological, Social and Biological Approaches to Schizophrenia*. Hove: Brunner-Routledge.

Reavley, N.J. and Jorm, A.F. (2011a) Recognition of mental disorders and beliefs about treatment and outcome: findings from an Australian National Survey of Mental Health Literacy and Stigma, *Australian and New Zealand Journal of Psychiatry*, 45: 947–956.

Reavley, N.J. and Jorm, A.F. (2011b) The quality of mental disorder information websites: a review, *Patient Education and Counselling*, 85: e16–e25.

Ricard, M. (2003) *Happiness: A Guide to Life's Most Important Skill*. New York: Little, Brown and Company.

Richter, L.M. (2006) Studying adolescence, *Science*, 312: 1902–1905.

Richter, L., Dawes, A. and de Kadt, J. (2010) Early childhood, in I. Petersen, A. Petersen, A. Bhana, A.J. Flisher, L. Swartz and L. Richter (eds), *Promoting Mental Health in Scarce-Resource Contexts. Emerging Evidence and Practice*. Cape Town: HSRC Press.

Ridley, M. (2003) *Nature via Nurture: Genes, Experience and What Makes Us Human*. London: HarperCollins.

Roberts, B. (2005) *The End of Oil*. London: Bloomsbury.

Robertson, I. and Cooper, C.L. (2011) *Wellbeing: Productivity and Happiness at Work*. London: Palgrave Macmillan.

Roe, D., Hasson-Ohayon, I., Derhi, O., Yanos, P.T. and Lysaker, P.H. (2010) Talking about life and finding solutions to different hardships: a qualitative study on the impact of narrative enhancement and cognitive therapy on persons with serious mental illness, *Journal of Nervous and Mental Disease*, 198: 807–812.

Rogers, A. and Pilgrim, D. (2003) *Inequalities and Mental Health*. London: Palgrave Macmillan.

Rones, M. and Hoagwood, K. (2000) School-based mental health services: a research review, *Clinical Child and Family Psychology Review*, 3: 223–241.

Rose, D. (2001) *Users' Voices: The Perspectives of Mental Health Service Users on Community and Hospital Care*. London: The Sainsbury Centre.

Rose, G. (1992) *The Strategy of Preventive Medicine*. Oxford: Oxford University Press.

Rosen, A. (2006). Destigmatizing day-to-day practices: what developed countries can learn from developing countries, *World Psychiatry*, 5: 21–24.

Rossler, W. (2006) Psychiatric rehabilitation today: an overview, *World Psychiatry*, 5: 151–157.

Roulstone, A. and Warren, J. (2005) Applying a barriers approach to monitoring disabled people's employ-ment: implications for the Disability Discrimination Act 2005, *Disability and Society*, 21: 115–131.

Rowling, L. (2002) Mental health promotion, in L. Rowling, G. Martin and L. Walker (eds), *Mental Health Promotion and Young People* (pp. 10–23). London: McGraw-Hill.

Rowling, L. and Weist, M.D. (2004) Promoting the growth, improvement and sustainability of school mental health programs worldwide, *International Journal of Mental Health Promotion*, 6: 3–11.

Rubin, H.J. and Rubin, S. (2008) *Community Organising and Development*, 4th edn. Boston, MA: Pearson.

Rudman, L.A., Ashmore, R.D. and Gary, M.L. (2001) 'Unlearning' automatic biases: The malleability of implicit prejudice and stereotypes, *Journal of Personality and Social Psychology*, 81: 856–88.

Rüsch, N., Hölzer, A., Hermann, C., Schramm, E., Jacob, G.A., Bohus, M., Lieb, K. and Corrigan, P.W. (2006) Self-stigma in women with borderline personality disorder and women with social phobia, *Journal of Nervous and Mental Disease*, 194: 766–773.

Rüsch, N., Corrigan, P.W., Powell, K., Rajah, A., Olschewski, M., Wilkniss, S. and Batia, K. (2009a) A stress-coping model of mental illness stigma: II. Emotional stress responses, coping behavior and outcome, *Schizophrenia Research*, 110: 65–71.

Rüsch, N., Corrigan, P.W., Wassel, A., Michaels, P., Larson, J.E., Olschewski, M., Wilkness, S. and Batia, K. (2009b) Self-stigma, group identification, perceived legitimacy of discrimination and mental health service use, *British Journal of Psychiatry*, 195: 551–552.

Rüsch, N., Corrigan, P.W., Wassel, A., Michaels, P., Olschewski, M., Wilkniss, S. and Batia, K. (2009c) Ingroup perception and responses to stigma among persons with mental illness, *Acta Psychiatrica Scandinavica*, 120: 320–328.

Rüsch, N., Todd, A.R., Bodenhausen, G.V., Weiden, P.J. and Corrigan, P.W. (2009d) Implicit versus explicit attitudes toward psychiatric medication: implications for insight and treatment adherence, *Schizophrenia Research*, 112: 119–122.

Rüsch, N., Corrigan, P.W., Todd, A.R. and Bodenhausen, G.V. (2010a) Implicit self-stigma in people with mental illness, *Journal of Nervous and Mental Disease*, 198: 150–153.

Rüsch, N., Todd, A.R., Bodenhausen, G.V. and Corrigan, P.W. (2010b) Biogenetic models of psychopathology, implicit guilt, and mental illness stigma, *Psychiatry Research*, 179: 328–332.

Rüsch, N., Todd, A.R., Bodenhausen, G.V. and Corrigan, P.W. (2010c). Do people with mental illness deserve what they get? Links between meritocratic worldviews and implicit versus explicit stigma, *European Archives of Psychiatry and Clinical Neurosciences*, 260: 617–625.

Rüsch, N., Todd, A.R., Bodenhausen, G.V., Olschewski, M. and Corrigan, P.W. (2010d) Automatically activated shame reactions and perceived legitimacy of discrimination: a longitudinal study among people with mental illness, *Journal of Behavior Therapy and Experimental Psychiatry*, 41: 60–63.

Rutherford, J. (2008) Cultures of capitalism, *Soundings*, 38: 8–18.

Ryan, R.M. and Deci, E.L. (2001) On happiness and human potentials: a review of research on hedonic and eudaimonic wellbeing, *Annual Reviews of Psychology*, 52: 141–166.

Ryff, C.D. (1989) Happiness is everything; or is it? Explorations on the meaning of psychological wellbeing, *Journal of Personality and Social Psychology*, 57: 1069–1081.

Ryff, C.D. and Keyes, C.L.M. (1995) The structure of psychological well-being revisited, *Journal of Personality and Social Psychology*, 69: 719–727.

Sainsbury Centre for Mental Health (2006) *The Future of Mental Health: A Vision for 2015*. London: The Sainsbury Centre.

Saleeby, D. (2006) *The Strengths Perspective in Social Work Practice*, 4th edn. Boston, MA: Allyn and Bacon.

Salokangas, R.K.R. and Poutanen, O. (1998) Risk factors for depression in primary care: findings of the TADEP project, *Journal of Affective Disorders*, 48: 171–180.

Salovey, P. and Sluyter. D.J. (1997) *Emotional Development and Emotional Intelligence: Educational Implications*. New York: Basic Books.

Samaritans (2012) *Suicide Statistics Report 2011*. Available at www.samaritans.org (accessed 20 January 2012).

Sanddal, N.D., Sanddal, T.L., Berman, A.L. and Silverman, M.M. (2003) A general systems approach to suicide prevention: lessons from cardiac prevention and control, *Suicide and Life-Threatening Behavior*, 33: 341–352.

Saraceno, B., Itzhak, L. and Kohn, R. (2005) The public mental health significance of research on socio-economic factors in schizophrenia and major depression, *World Psychiatry*, 4: 181–185.

Sartorius, N. (2002) Iatrogenic stigma of mental illness, *British Medical Journal*, 324: 1470–1471.

Sartorius, N. and Schulze, H. (2005) *Reducing the Stigma of Mental Illness: A Report from a Global Association*. Cambridge: Cambridge University Press.

Saxena, S., Thornicroft, G., Knapp, M. and Whiteford, H. (2007) Resources for mental health: scarcity, inequity, and inefficiency, *Lancet*, 370: 878–889.

Sayce, L. (2000) *From Psychiatric Patient to Citizen*. London: Macmillan.

Scales, P. and Leffert, N. (1999) *Developmental Assets: A Synthesis of Scientific Research on Adolescent Development*. Minneapolis, MN: Search Institute.

Scharf, T. and De Jong Gierveld, J. (2008) Loneliness in urban neighbourhoods: an Anglo-Dutch comparison, *European Journal of Ageing*, 5: 103–115.

Schipperijn, J., Stigsdotter, U.K., Randrup, T. and Troelsen, J. (2010) Influences on the use of urban green space: a case study in Odense, Denmark, *Urban Forestry and Urban Greening*, 9: 25–32.

Schomerus, G. and Angermeyer, M.C. (2008) Stigma and its impact on help-seeking for mental disorders: what do we know?, *Epidemiologia e Psichiatria Sociale*, 17: 31–37.

Schomerus, G., Angermeyer, M.C., Matschinger, H. and Riedel-Heller, S.G. (2008) Public attitudes towards prevention of depression, *Journal of Affective Disorders*, 106: 257–263.

Schore, A. (2001) The effects of early relational trauma on right brain development, affect regulation, and infant mental health, *Infant Mental Health Journal*, 22: 201–269.

Schwartz, B. (2000) Self-determination: the tyranny of freedom, *American Psychologist*, 55: 79–88.

Schwartz, B. (2004) *The Paradox of Choice*. New York: HarperCollins.

Scottish Government, The (2009) *Towards a Mentally Flourishing Scotland*. Edinburgh: Scottish Government.

Seligman, M. (2002) *Authentic Happiness: Using the Power of Positive Psychology to Realize your Potential for Lasting Fulfilment*. New York: The Free Press.

Semmer, N.K. (2008) Stress management and wellbeing interventions in the workplace, in J.M. Kidd (ed.), *Mental Capital and Wellbeing: Making the Most of Ourselves in the 21st Century*. London: Government Office for Science.

Sen, A. (1988) Freedom of choice, concept and content, *European Economic Review*, 32: 269–298.

Sennett, R. (2006) *The Culture of the New Capitalism*. New Haven, CN: Yale University Press.

Shemmings, D. and Shemmings, Y. (2011) *Understanding Disorganised Attachment. Theory and Practice for Working with Children and Adults*. London: Jessica Kingsley Publisher.

Shi, L., Starfield, B., Politzer, R. and Regan, J. (2002 Primary care, self-rated health, and reductions in social disparities in health, *Health Services Research*, 37: 529–550.

Shorter, E. (1997) *A History of Psychiatry: From the Era of the Asylum to the Age of Prozac*. New York: Wiley.

Shutte, N.S., Malouff, J.M., Hall, L.E., Haggerty, D.J., Cooper, J.T., Golden, C.J. and Dornheim, L. (1998) Development and validation of a measure of emotional intelligence, *Personality and Individual Differences*, 25: 167–177.

Simonsen, E., Friis, S., Opjordsmoen, S., Mortensen, E.L., Haahr, U., Melle, I., Joa, I., Johannessen, J.O., Larsen, T.K., Røssberg, J.I., Rund, B.R., Vaglum, P. and McGlashan, T.H. (2010) Early identification of non-remission in first-episode psychosis in a two-year outcome study, *Acta Psychiatrica Scandanavica*, 122: 375–383.

Singer, B. and Ryff, C. (eds) (2001) *New Horizons in Health: An Integrative Approach*. Washington DC: National Academies Press.

Slade, A., Grienenberger, J., Bernbach, E., Levy, D. and Locker, A. (2001) *Maternal Reflective Functioning: Considering the Transmission Gap*. Paper presented at the Biennial Meeting of the Society for Research in Child Development, Minneapolis, MN.

Slade, M. (2010) Mental illness and well-being: the central importance of positive psychology and recovery approaches, *BMC Health Services Research*, 10: 26.

Sobocki, P., Jonsson, B., Angst, J. and Rehnberg, C. (2006) Cost of depression in Europe, *Journal of Mental Health Policy Economics*, 9: 87–98.

Social Exclusion Unit (2004) *Mental Health and Social Exclusion*. London: Office of the Deputy Prime Minister.

Social Exclusion Unit (2006) *A Sure Start to Later Life: Ending Inequalities for Older People*. London: Office of the Deputy Prime Minister.

Soule, A., Babb, P., Evandrou, M., Balchin, S. and Zealey, L. (2005) *Focus on Older People*. London: National Statistics.

Sperber, E., Mckay, M.M., Bell, C.C., Petersen, I., Bhana, A. and Paikoff, R. (2008) Adapting and disseminating a community-collaborative, evidence-based HIV/AIDS prevention programme: lessons from the history of CHAMP, *Vulnerable Children and Youth Studies*, 3: 150–158.

Spitzer, R.L., Kroenke, K. and Williams, J.B.W. (1999) Validation and utility of a self-report version of PRIME-MD: the PHQ primary care study. Primary Care Evaluation of Mental Disorders. Patient Health Questionnaire, *Journal of the American Medical Association*, 282: 1737–1744.

Spreitzer, G. and Porath, C. (2012) Creating sustainable performance, *Harvard Business Review*, January–February: 92–99.

Sroufe, L.A. (1996) *Emotional Development: The Organization of Emotional Life in the Early Years*. New York: Cambridge University Press.

Sroufe, L.A. (2005) Attachment and development: a prospective, longitudinal study from birth to adulthood, *Attachment and Human Development*, 7: 349–367.

Stackert, R.A. and Bursik, K. (2003) Why am I unsatisfied? Adult attachment style, gendered irrational relationship beliefs, and young adult romantic relationship satisfaction, *Personality and Individual Differences*, 34: 1419–1429.

Stansfeld, S.A., Fuhrer, R., Shipley, M.J. and Marmot, M.G. (1999) Work characteristics predict psychiatric disorder: prospective results from the Whitehall II Study, *Occupational and Environmental Medicine*, 56: 302–307.

Staup, J. (1999) *The Integration of Mental Health and Education Systems*. Presented at the Fourth National Conference on Advancing School-Based Mental Health Programs, Denver, CO.

Steele, H. and Steele, M. (2008) On the origins of reflective functioning, in F. Busch (ed.), *Mentalization: Theoretical Considerations, Research Findings and Clinical Implications*. New York: Taylor and Francis.

Stephan, S.H., Mulloy, M. and Brey, L. (2011) Improving collaborative mental health care by school-based primary care and mental health providers, *School Mental Health*, 3: 70–80.

Stewart-Brown, S. (2002) Measuring the parts most measures do not reach: a necessity for evaluation in mental health promotion, *Journal of Mental Health Promotion*, 1: 4–9.

Stewart-Brown, S. (2013) The Warwick Edinburgh Mental Well-being Scale (WEMWBS): performance in different cultural and geographical groups, in C. Keyes (ed.), *Mental Well-Being: International Contributions to the Study of Positive Mental Health*. New York: Springer.

Stewart-Brown, S., Tennant, A., Tennant, R., Platt, S., Parkinson, J. and Weich, S. (2009) Internal construct validity of the Warwick-Edinburgh Mental Well-being Scale (WEMWBS): a Rasch analysis using data from the Scottish Health Education Population Survey, *Health and Quality of Life Outcomes*, 7: 15.

Stiglitz, J.E., Sen, A. and Fitoussi, J.P. (2009) *Report by the Commission on Measurement of Economic and Social Progress*. Available at http://www.stiglitz-sen-fitoussi.fr/en/index.htm (accessed 22 August 2012).

Stroul, B. (2007) *Integrating Mental Health Services into Primary Care Settings – Summary of the Special Forum at the 2006 Georgetown University Training Institutes*. Washington, DC: Georgetown University Center for Child and Human Development, National Technical Assistance Center for Children's Mental Health.

Stuart, H. (2006) Mental illness and employment discrimination, *Current Opinion in Psychiatry*, 19, 522–526.

Stuckler, D., Basu, S., Suhrcke, M., Coutts, A. and McKee, M. (2011) Effects of the 2008 recession on health: a first look at European data, *Lancet*, 378: 124–125.

Subramanian, D.N. and Hopayian, K. (2008) An audit of the first year of screening for depression in patients with diabetes and ischaemic heart disease under the Quality and Outcomes Framework, *Quality in Primary Care*, 16: 341–344.

Subramanian, S.V. and Kawachi, I. (2004) Income inequality and health: what have we learned so far?, *Epidemiological Review*, 26: 78–91.

Suchman, N., DeCoste, C., Castiglioni, N., Legow, N. and Mayes, L. (2008) The Mothers and Toddlers Program: preliminary findings from an attachment-based parenting intervention for substance-abusing mothers, *Psychoanalytic Psychology*, 25: 499–517.

Suchman, N.E., DeCoste, C., Castiglioni, N., McMahon, T.J., Rounsaville, B. and Mayes, L. (2010) The Mothers and Toddlers Program, an attachment-based parenting intervention for substance using women: post-treatment results from a randomized clinical pilot, *Attachment and Human Development*, 12: 483–504.

Sugai, G. and Horner, R.H. (2002) The evolution of discipline practices: school-wide positive behavior supports, *Child and Family Behavior Therapy*, 24: 23–25.

Sugai, G., Horner, R.H., Dunlap, G., Hieneman, M., Lewis, T.J., Nelson, C.M., Scott, T., Liaupsin, C., Sailor, W., Turnbull, A.P., Turnbull, H.R., III, Wickham, D., Reuf, M. and Wilcox, B. (2000) Applying positive behavioral support and functional behavioral assessment in schools, *Journal of Positive Behavioral Interventions*, 2: 131–143.

ten Have, M., de Graaf, R., Ormel, J., Vilagut, G., Kovess, V. and Alonso, J. (2009) Are attitudes towards mental health help-seeking associated with service use? Results from the European Study of Epidemiology of Mental Disorders, *Social Psychiatry and Psychiatric Epidemiology*, 45: 153–163.

Tennant, R., Hiller, L., Fishwick, R., Platt, P., Joseph, S., Weich, S., Parkinson, J., Secker, J. and Stewart-Brown, S. (2007a). The Warwick-Edinburgh Mental Well-being Scale (WEMWBS): development and UK validation, *Health and Quality of Life Outcomes*, 5: 63.

Tennant, R., Joseph, S. and Stewart-Brown, S. (2007b) The Affectometer 2: a valid measure of positive mental health in UK populations, *Quality of Life Research*, 16: 687–695.

The Government Office for Science (2008) *Mental Capital and Wellbeing: Making the Most of Ourselves in the 21st Century*. London: The Government Office for Science.

Thombs, B.D., Coyne, J.C., Cuijpers, P., de Jonge, P., Gilbody, S., Ioannidis, J.P., Johnson, B.T., Patten, S.B., Turner, E.H. and Ziegelstein, R.C. (2011) Rethinking recommendations for screening for depression in primary care, *Canadian Medical Association Journal*, 184: 413–418.

Thompson, A., Issakidis, C.N. and Hunt, C. (2008) Delay to seek treatment for anxiety and mood disorders in an Australian clinical sample, *Behaviour Change*, 25: 71–84.

Thomson, H. and Petticrew, M. (2005) *Is Housing Improvement a Potential Health Improvement Strategy?* Geneva: WHO Europe Health Evidence Network.

Thomson, H., Atkinson, R., Petticrew, M. and Kearns, A. (2006) Do urban regeneration programmes improve public health and reduce health inequalities? A synthesis of the evidence from UK policy and practice (1980–2004), *Journal of Epidemiology and Community Health*, 60: 108–115.

Thornicroft, G. (2006) *Shunned: Discrimination against People with Mental Illness*. Oxford: Oxford University Press.

Thornicroft, G., Brohan, E., Kassam, A. and Lewis-Holmes, E. (2008) Reducing stigma and discrimination: candidate interventions, *International Journal of Mental Health Systems*, 2: 3.

Thornicroft, G., Brohan, E., Rose, D., Sartorius, N. and Leese, M. (2009) Global pattern of experienced and anticipated discrimination against people with schizophrenia: a cross-sectional survey, *Lancet*, 373: 408–415.

Timonen, M. and Liukkonen, T. (2008) Management of depression in adults, *British Medical Journal*, 336: 435–439.

Tognoni, G., Alli, C., Avanzini, F., Bettelli, G., Colombo. F., Corso, R., Marchioli, R. and Zussino, A. (1991) Randomised clinical trials in general practice: lessons from a failure, *British Medical Journal*, 303: 969–971.

Tomlinson, M. and Landman, M. (2007) 'It's not just about food': mother-infant interaction and the wider context of nutrition, *Maternal and Child Nutrition*, 3: 292–302.

Tooth, B., Kalyanansundaram, V. and Glover, H. (1997) *Recovery from Schizophrenia: A Consumer Perspective. Final Report to Health and Human Services Research and Development Grants Program (RADGAC)*. Queensland: Centre for Mental Health Nursing Research.

Tourangeau, R. and Smith, T.W. (1996) Asking sensitive questions: the impact of data collection mode, question format, and question context, *Public Opinion Quarterly*, 60: 275–304.

Tudor Hart, J. (1971) The inverse care law, *Lancet*, i: 405–412.

Tudor, K. (1996) *Mental Health Promotion: Paradigms and Practice*. London: Routledge.

Turner, K.M., Sharp, D., Folkes, L. and Chew-Graham, C. (2008) Women's views and experiences of anti-depressants as a treatment for postnatal depression: a qualitative study, *Family Practice*, 25: 450–455.

Twelvetrees, A. (2008) *Community Work*, 4th edn. Basingstoke: Palgrave MacMillan.

United Nations Children's Fund (2007) *Child Poverty in Perspective: An Overview of Child Wellbeing in Rich Countries*. Florence: UNICEF.

United Nations Office on Drugs and Crime (2007) *World Drug Report*. Vienna: UN Office on Drugs and Crime.

US Department of Health and Human Services (1999) *Mental Health: A Report of the Surgeon General*. Rockville, MD: US Department of Health and Human Services, National Institute of Mental Health.

van Ijzendoorn, M.H. and Sagi, A. (1999) Cross-cultural patterns of attachment: Universal and contextual dimensions, in J. Cassidy and P. Shaver (eds), *Handbook of Attachment*. New York: Guilford.

van Ijzendoorn, M.H., Schuengel, C. and Bakermans-Kranenburg, M. (1999) Disorganized attachment in early childhood: meta-analysis of precursors, concomitants, and sequelae, *Development and Psychopathology*, 11: 225–250.

van Os, V., Pedersen, C.B. and Mortensen, P.B. (2004) Confirmation of the synergy between urbanicity and familial liability in the causation of psychosis, *American Journal of Psychiatry*, 161:2312–2314.

Vaughan, G. and Hansen, C. (2004) 'Like minds, like mine': a New Zealand project to counter the stigma and discrimination associated with mental illness, *Australasian Psychiatry*, 12: 113–117.

Velasquez, M. (2009) *Philosophy: A Text with Readings*, 11th edn: 120. Boston, MA: Wadsworth.

Victor, C., Scambler, S. and Bond, J. (2009) *The Social World of Older People: Understanding Loneliness and Social Isolation in Later Life*. Maidenhead: Open University Press/McGraw-Hill.

von Bonsdorff, M.B. and Rantanen, T. (2010) Benefits of formal voluntary work among older people. A review, *Aging Clinical and Experimental Research*, 23: 162–169.

Von Korff, M. and Goldberg, D. (2001) Improving outcomes in depression, *British Medical Journal*, 323: 948–949.

Waddell, G. and Burton, A.K. (2006) *Is Work Good for Your Health and Well-being?* Norwich: The Stationery Office.

Wahl, O.F. (1995) *Media Madness: Public Images of Mental Illness*. New Brunswick, NJ: Rutgers University Press.

Walker, J. (2008) Communication and social work from an attachment perspective, *Journal of Social Work Practice*, 22: 5–13.

Walker, S.P., Chang, S.M., Powell, C.A., Simonoff, E. and Grantham-McGregor, S. (2007a) Early childhood stunting is associated with poor psychological functioning in late adolescence and effects are reduced by psychosocial stimulation, *Journal of Nutrition*, 137: 2464–2469.

Walker, S.P., Wachs, T.D., Gardner, J.M., Lozoff, B., Wasserman, G.A., Pollitt, E. and Carter, J.A. (2007b) Child development: risk factors for adverse outcomes in developing countries, *Lancet*, 369: 145–157.

Walker, S.P., Chang, S.M., Vera-Hernández, M. and Grantham-McGregor, S. (2011) Early childhood stimulation benefits adult competence and reduces violent behavior, *Pediatrics*, 127: 849–857.

Wallcraft, J. (2009) *Recovery – A Double Edged Sword?* Paper presented at Critical Psychiatry Network Conference 2009. Available at ww.mentalhealth.freeuk.com/Doubleedged.htm (accessed 24 August 2012).

Wallerstein, N. (2006) *What is the Evidence on Effectiveness of Empowerment to Improve Health?* Geneva: WHO Europe Health Evidence Network.

Walsh, B.T., Seidman, S.N., Sysko, R. and Gould, M. (2002) Placebo response in studies of major depression variable, substantial, and growing, *Journal of the American Medical Association*, 287: 1840–1847.

Wang, J., Adair, C., Fick, G., Lai, D., Evans, B., Perry, B.W., Jorm, A. and Addington, D. (2007b) Depression literacy in Alberta: findings from a general population sample, *Canadian Journal of Psychiatry*, 52: 442–449.

Wang, P.S., Simon, G. and Kessler, R.C. (2003) The economic burden of depression and the cost-effectiveness of treatment, *International Journal of Methods in Psychiatric Research*, 12: 22–33.

Wang, P.S., Aguilar-Gaxiola, S., Alonso, J., Angermeyer, M.C., Borges, G., Bromet, E.J., Bruffaerts, R., de Girolamo, G., de Graaf, R., Gureje, O., Haro, J.M., Karam, E.G., Kessler, R.C., Kovess, V., Lane, M.C., Lee, S., Levinson, D., Ono, Y., Petukhova, M., Posada-Villa, J., Seedat, S. and Wells, J.E. (2007) Use of mental health services for anxiety, mood, and substance disorders in 17 countries in the WHO world mental health surveys, *Lancet*, 370: 841–850.

Wang, P.S., Angermeyer, M., Borges, G., Bruffaerts, R., Tat Chiu, W., De Girolamo, G., Fayyad, J., Gureje, O., Haro, J.M., Huang, Y., Kessler, R.C., Kovess, V., Levinson, D., Nakane, Y., Oakley Brown, M.A., Ormel, J.H., Posada-Villa, J., Aguilar-Gaxiola, S., Alonso, J., Lee, S., Heeringa, S., Pennell, B.E., Chatterji, S. and Üstün, T.B. (2007a) Delay and failure in treatment seeking after first onset of mental disorders in the World Health Organization's World Mental Health Survey Initiative, *World Psychiatry*, 6: 177–185.

Warner, R. (2004) *Recovery from Schizophrenia: Psychiatry and Political Economy*. New York: Routledge.

Wasserman, D. and Wasserman, C. (eds) (2009) *Oxford Textbook of Suicidology and Suicide Prevention*. Oxford: Oxford University Press.

Watson, D., Clark, L.A. and Tellegen, A. (1988) Development and validation of brief measures of positive and negative affect: the PANAS scales, *Journal of Personality and Social Psychology*, 6: 1063–1070.

Waxman, R.P., Weist, M.D. and Benson, D.M. (1999) Toward collaboration in the growing education-mental health interface, *Clinical Psychology Review*, 19: 239–253.

Wedding, D. and Mengel, M. (2004) Models of integrated care in primary care setting, in L.J. Haas (ed.), *Handbook of Primary Care Psychology*: 47–60. New York: Oxford University Press.

Weich, S. and Lewis, G. (1998) Material standard of living, social class, and the prevalence of the common mental disorders in Great Britain, *Journal of Epidemiology and Community Health*, 52: 8–14.

Weich, S., Lewis, G. and Jenkins, S.P. (2001) Income inequality and the prevalence of common mental disorders in Britain, *British Journal of Psychiatry*, 178: 222–227.

Weich, S., Brugha, T., King, M., McManus, S., Bebbington, P., Jenkins, R., Cooper, C., McBride, O. and Stewart-Brown, S. (2011) Mental well-being and mental illness: Findings from the adult psychiatric morbidity survey for England 2007, *British Journal of Psychiatry*, 199: 23–28.

Weiss, C.H. (1995) Nothing as practical as good theory: exploring theory-based evaluation for comprehensive community initiatives for children and families, in J.P. Connell, A.C. Kubish, L.B. Schorr and C.H. Weiss (eds), *New Approaches to Evaluating Community Initiatives. Volume 1: Concepts, Methods and Contexts*. Washington DC: Aspen Institute.

Weist, M.D. (1997) Expanded school mental health services: a national movement in progress, in T. Ollendick and R. J. Prinz (eds), *Advanced Clinical Child Psycholog (Vol. 19)*: 319–352. New York: Plenum Press.

Weist, M. (2005) Fulfilling the promise of school-based mental health: moving toward a public mental health promotion approach, *Journal of Abnormal Clinical Psychology*, 33: 735–741.

Weist, M. and Ghuman, H. (2002) Principles behind the proactive delivery of mental health services to youth where they are, in H. Ghuman, M.D. Wiest and R. Sarles (eds), *Providing Mental Health Services Where They Are: School and Community-Based Approaches*. New York: Taylor and Francis.

Weist, M.D. and Murray, M. (2007) Advancing school mental health promotion globally, *Advances in School Mental Health Promotion*, Inaugural Issue: 2–12.

Weist, M.D., and Rowling, L. (2002) International efforts to advance mental health in schools, *International Journal of Mental Health Promotion*, 4: 3–7.

Weist, M.D., Sander, M.A., Nabors, L.A., Link, B. and Christodulu, K.V. (2002) Advancing the quality agenda in expanded school mental health, *Emotional and Behavioral Disorders in Youth*, 2, 59–63.

Weist, M.D., Goldstein, J., Evans, S.W., Lever, N.A., Axelrod, J., Schreters, R. and Pruitt, D. (2003) Funding a full continuum of mental health promotion and intervention programs in the schools, *Journal of Adolescent Health*, 32: 70–78.

Weist, M.D., Lever, N., Stephan, S., Youngstrom, E., Moore, E., Harrison, B., Anthony, L., Rogers, K., Hoagwood, K., Ghunney, A., Lewis, K. and Stiegler, K. (2009) Formative evaluation of a framework for high quality, evidence-based services in school mental health, *School Mental Health*, 1: 196–211.

Wells, J.E., Oakely-Brown, M.A., Scott, K.M., Mcgee, M.A., Baxter, J., Kokaua, J.; New Zealand Mental Health Survey Research Team (2006) Te Rau Hinengaro: the New Zealand Mental Health Survey: overview of methods and findings, *Australian and New Zealand Journal of Psychiatry*, 40: 835–844.

Wenger, E. (1998) *Communities of Practice: Learning, Meaning and Identity*. New York: Cambridge University Press.

Whooley, M.A., Avins, A.L., Miranda, J. and Browner, W.S. (1997) Case-finding instruments for depression: two questions are as good as many, *Journal of General Internal Medicine*, 12: 439–445.

Wilkinson, R.G.(2005) *The Impact of Inequality: How to Make Sick Societies Healthier*. New York: The New Press.

Wilkinson, R.G. and Marmot, M. (2003) *Social Determinants of Health: The Solid Facts*, 2nd edn. Copenhagen: World Health Organization Europe.

Wilkinson, R.G. and Pickett, K.E. (2006) Income inequality and population health: a review and explanation of the evidence, *Social Science and Medicine*, 62: 1768–1784.

Wilkinson, R.G. and Pickett, K.E. (2007) The problems of relative deprivation: why some societies do better than others, *Social Science and Medicine*, 65: 1965–1978.

Wilkinson, R.G. and Pickett, K.E. (2009a) Income inequality and social dysfunction, *Annual Review of Sociology*, 35: 493–511.

Wilkinson, R.G. and Pickett, K.E. (2009b) *The Sprit Level: Why More Equal Societies Almost Always do Better*. London: Allen Lane.

Wilkinson, R.G. and Pickett, K.E. (2010) *The Spirit Level: Why Equality is Better for Everyone*. London: Penguin.

Williams, S.J. (2000) Reason, emotion and embodiment: is 'mental' health a contradiction in terms? *Sociology of Health and Illness*, 22: 559–581.

Wilson, S., Delaney, B.C., Roalfe, A., Roberts, L., Redman, V., Wearn, A.M. and Hobbs, F.D. (2000) Randomised controlled trials in primary care: case study, *British Medical Journal*, 321: 24–27.

Wilson, T.D. (2002) *Strangers to Ourselves: Exploring the Adaptive Unconscious*. Cambridge, MA: Harvard University Press.

Wilson, D.B., Gottfredson, D.C. and Najaka, S.S. (2001) School-based prevention of problem behaviors: a meta-analysis, *Journal of Quantitative Criminology*, 17: 247–272.

Windle, G., Hughes, D.A., Linck, P., Russell, I.T. and Woods, R.T. (2010) Is exercise effective in promoting mental well-being in older age? A systematic review, *Aging and Mental Health*, 14: 652–669.

Wittenbrink, B. (2007) Measuring attitudes through priming, in B. Wittenbrink and N. Schwarz (eds), *Implicit Measures of Attitudes* (pp. 17–58). New York: Guilford Press.

Wolfson, M., Kaplan, G., Lynch, J., Ross, N. and Backlund, E. (1999) Relation between income inequality and mortality: empirical demonstration, *British Medical Journal*, 319: 953–955.

World Economic Forum (2010a) *The New Discipline of Workforce Wellness: Enhancing Corporate Performance by Tackling Chronic Disease*. Geneva: World Economic Forum.

World Economic Forum (2010b) *The Wellness Imperative – Creating More Effective Organizations*. Geneva: World Economic Forum.

World Economic Forum (2011) *Wellness Alliance for Workplace Health*. Geneva: World Economic Forum.

World Economic Forum (2012). *The Workplace Wellness Alliance: Investing in a Sustainable Workforce*. Geneva: World Economic Forum. Available at www3.weforum.org/docs/WEF_HE_WorkplaceWellnessAlliance_IndustryAgenda_2012.pdf (accessed 1 October 2012).

World Health Organization (2001) *The World Health Report 2001. Mental Health: New Understanding, New Hope*. Geneva: WHO.

World Health Organization (2001a) *Mental Health: New Understanding, New Hope*. Geneva: WHO.

World Health Organization (2001b) *Strengthening Mental Health Promotion (Fact sheet No 220)*. Geneva: WHO.

World Health Organization (2003) *Caring for Children and Adolescents with Mental Health Disorders: Setting WHO Directions*. Geneva: WHO.

World Health Organization (2004a) *Promoting Mental Health. Concepts, Emerging Evidence, Practice. Summary Report*. Geneva: WHO.

World Health Organization (2004b) *The Global Burden of Disease*. Geneva: WHO.

World Health Organization (2005) *Promoting Mental Health: Concepts, Emerging Evidence, Practice*. Geneva: WHO.

World Health Organization (2008) *Global Burden of Disease 2004 Update*. Geneva: WHO.

World Health Organization (2008) *Global Burden of Disease*. Geneva: World Health Organization.

World Health Organization (2010) *Mental Health and Well-being at the Workplace – Protection and Inclusion in Challenging Times*. Copenhagen: WHO Europe.

World Health Organization (2010a) *mhGAP Intervention Guide*. Geneva: WHO.

World Health Organization (2010b) *Preventing Intimate Partner and Sexual Violence against Women: Taking Action and Generating Evidence*. Geneva: WHO.

World Health Organization (2011a) *Definition of an Older or Elderly Person*. Geneva: WHO. Available at www.who.int/healthinfo/survey/ageingdefnolder/en/index.html (accessed 28 August 2012).

World Health Organization (2011b) *What is Mental Health?* Geneva: WHO. Available at www.who.int/features/qa/62/en/index.html (accessed 28 August 2012).

World Health Organization (2011c) *What is Active Ageing?* Geneva: WHO. Available at www.who.int/ageing/active_ageing/en/index.html (accessed 5 December 2011).

World Health Organization (2012) *Suicide Prevention Reports*. Available at www.who.int/mental_health/prevention/suicide/suicideprevent/en (accessed 21 August 2012).

World Health Organization and the Commission on Social Determinants of Health (2008) *Closing the Gap in a Generation: Health Equity through Action on the Social Determinants of Health*. Geneva: WHO Publications.

World Health Organization and World Economic Forum (2008) *Preventing Noncommunicable Diseases in the Workplace through Diet and Physical Activity*. Geneva: WHO/World Economic Forum.

World Health Organization International Consortium in Psychiatric Epidemiology (2000) Cross-national comparisons of the prevalence and correlates of mental disorders, *Bulletin of the World Health Organization*, 78: 413–426.

Wright, A. and Jorm, A.F. (2009) Labels used by young people to describe mental disorders: factors associated with their development, *Australian and New Zealand Journal of Psychiatry*, 43: 946–955.

Wright, A., Harris, M.G., Wiggers, J.H., Jorm, A.F., Cotton, S.M., Harrigan, S.M., Hurworth, R.E. and McGorry, P.D. (2005) Recognition of depression and psychosis by young Australians and their beliefs about treatment, *Medical Journal of Australia*, 183: 18–23.

Wright, A., McGorry, P.D., Harris, M.G., Jorm, A.F. and Pennell, K. (2006) Development and evaluation of a youth mental health community awareness campaign – The Compass Strategy, *BMC Public Health*, 6: 215.

Wright, A., Jorm, A.F., Harris, M.G. and McGorry, P.D. (2007) What's in a name? Is accurate recognition and labelling of mental disorders by young people associated with better help-seeking and treatment preferences?, *Social Psychiatry and Psychiatric Epidemiology*, 42: 244–250.

Yap, M.B.H., Wright, A. and Jorm, A.F. (2011) First aid actions taken by young people for mental disorders in a close friend or family member: findings from an Australian national survey of youth, *Psychiatry Research*, 188: 123–128.

Zahran, H.S., Kobau, R., Moriarty, D.G., Zack, M.M., Holt, J. and Donehoo, R. (2005) Health-related quality of life surveillance–United States, 1993–2002, *Morbidity and Mortality Weekly Report Surveillance Summary*, 54: 1–35.

Zigmond, A.S. and Snaith, R.P. (1983) The Hospital Anxiety and Depression Scale, *Acta Psychiatrica Scandinavica*, 67: 361–370.

Zins, J.E. and Elias, M.E. (2006) Social and emotional learning, in G.G. Bear and K.M. Minke (eds), *Children's Needs III* (pp. 1–13). Bethesda, MD: National Association of School Psychologists.

Zins, J.E., Bloodworth, M.R., Weissberg, R.P. and Walhberg, H.J. (2004) The scientific base linking social and emotional learning to school success, in J. Zins, R. Weissberg, M. Wang and H.L. Walberg (eds), *Building Academic Success on Social and Emotional Learning: What does the Research Say?*: 3–22. New York: Teachers College Press.

Index